DIABETIC DIET COOKBOOK AFTER 50

The Complete Nutrition Guide with 50 Quick and Easy Low-Sugar & Low-Carb Nutritious Recipes for Diabetes Management in Seniors

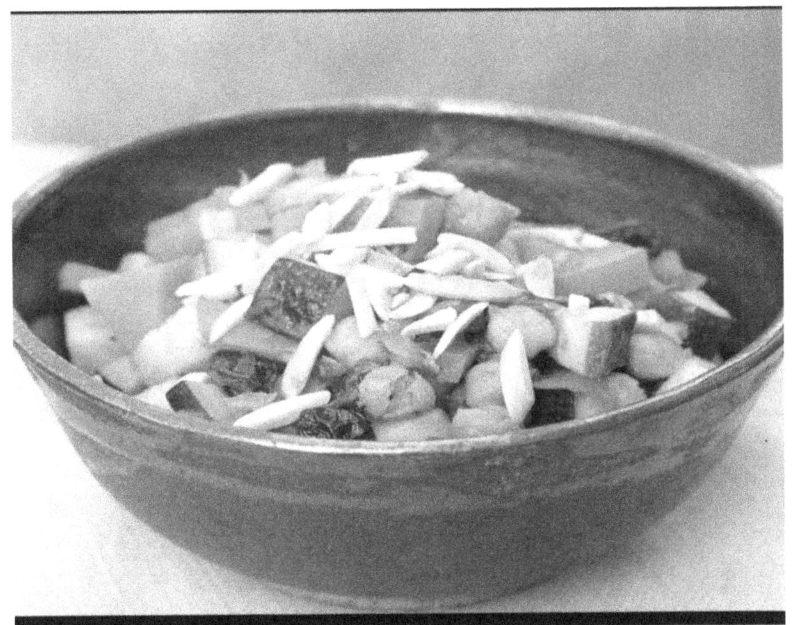

DR. COLE HULL

COPYRIGHT

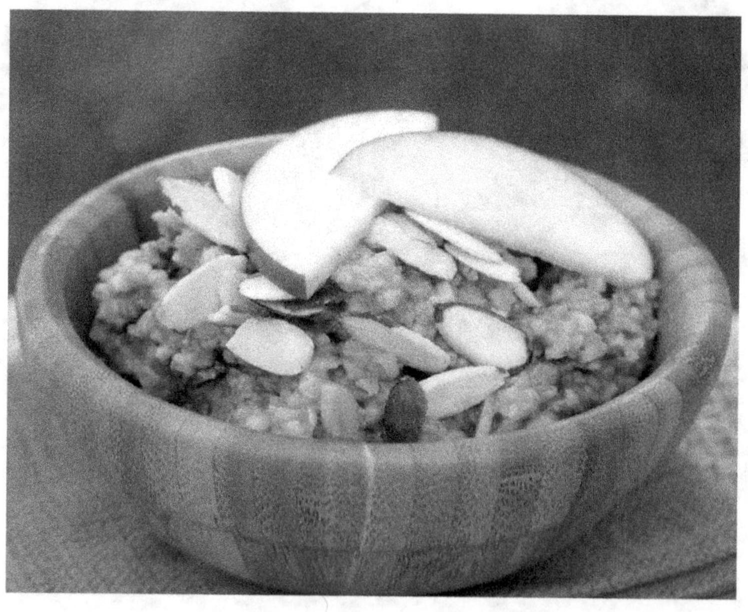

TABLE OF CONTENT

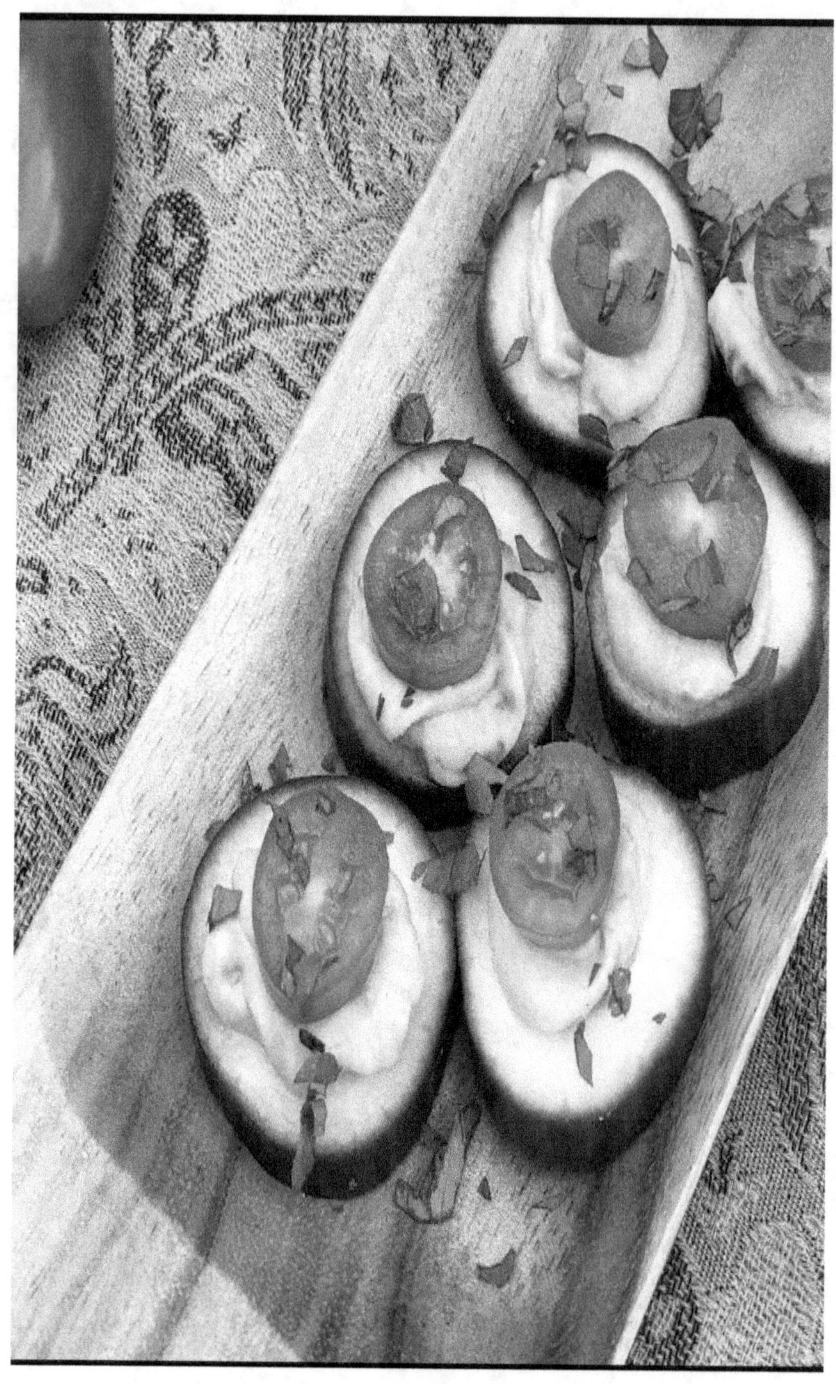

1. INTRODUCTION

Diabetes is a condition that becomes increasingly prevalent and complex with age. As individuals cross the age of 50, the risk of developing type 2 diabetes increases significantly due to various factors such as a sedentary lifestyle, weight gain, and changes in insulin sensitivity. For those already living with diabetes, the challenges are multifaceted, including managing blood sugar levels, dealing with potential complications, and making lifestyle adjustments.

This book, "Diabetic Diets Cookbook After 50," is designed to be your companion in navigating these challenges. It's not just about recipes; it's about understanding diabetes in the later stages of life and making informed decisions that can significantly improve your health and quality of life.

The journey through this book will equip you with the knowledge and tools necessary to manage diabetes effectively. You'll discover not only delicious and nutritious recipes but also gain insights into how your dietary choices impact your blood sugar levels and overall well-being.

Understanding Diabetes After 50

Diabetes after 50 presents unique challenges. At this age, the body's ability to produce and use insulin—the hormone that regulates blood sugar levels—can decrease. This change increases the risk of high blood sugar levels, a hallmark of diabetes. Additionally, age-related factors such as reduced physical activity, muscle loss, and increased body fat contribute to diabetes risk.

However, it's not just about the physical changes. The psychological and social aspects of managing diabetes after 50 are equally crucial. It may involve coping with other age-related health issues, adapting to lifestyle changes, and maintaining a healthy mental state.

Understanding these changes and challenges is the first step in managing diabetes effectively. This knowledge empowers you to make informed decisions about your diet, exercise, and overall lifestyle to keep your blood sugar levels in check and reduce the risk of complications.

With this understanding, we can appreciate why diet plays a pivotal role in managing diabetes, especially after the age of 50.

Importance of Diet in Managing Diabetes

The role of diet in managing diabetes, especially for those over 50, cannot be overstated. Proper nutrition is a cornerstone of diabetes management, as it directly impacts blood sugar levels, body weight, and overall health. A well-planned diet can help stabilize blood sugar, reduce the risk of complications, and even lessen the need for medication in some cases.

1. Blood Sugar Control: The primary goal in managing diabetes is to maintain healthy blood sugar levels. The foods you eat have a direct impact on glucose levels. Carbohydrates, in particular, break down into glucose and can cause blood sugar spikes if not managed correctly. Understanding which foods to eat, in what quantities, and when, is crucial for keeping your blood sugar within target ranges.

2. Weight Management: Many individuals over 50 struggle with weight control, which can be a significant risk factor for developing type 2 diabetes or exacerbating existing diabetes. A balanced diet helps in maintaining a healthy weight, reducing the strain on your body's ability to use insulin effectively.

3. Preventing Complications: Diabetes can lead to several complications, including heart disease, kidney damage, and vision problems. A nutritious diet, rich in fruits, vegetables, whole grains, lean proteins, and healthy fats, can help reduce the risk of these complications. It's also essential to limit foods high in sugar, unhealthy fats, and sodium.

4. Overall Well-being: Beyond managing blood sugar and preventing complications, a healthy diet contributes to better energy levels, improved mood, and enhanced cognitive function. This holistic approach is especially important as you age, ensuring not just a longer life, but a better quality of life.

In the subsequent chapters, we will explore specific foods and recipes that align with these dietary goals. You will learn how to enjoy delicious meals while also taking care of your health, proving that a diabetic diet after 50 can be both nutritious and enjoyable.

2. THE BASICS OF DIABETIC DIET

A diabetic diet is more than just a list of foods to eat and avoid; it's a balanced approach to eating that is tailored to your individual health needs, especially as you age. For those over 50 with diabetes, it's crucial to understand how foods affect blood sugar levels and overall health. This section of "Diabetic Diets Cookbook After 50" aims to provide a foundation for understanding the basics of a diabetic diet and how it can be adapted to the unique nutritional needs of older adults.

Nutritional Needs for Over 50s with Diabetes

As you age, your body's nutritional needs change, and managing diabetes adds another layer of consideration. Here are key nutritional aspects to focus on:

1. Lower Caloric Needs: Metabolism slows down as you age, reducing your caloric requirements. It's important to focus on nutrient-dense foods that provide the necessary vitamins and minerals without excessive calories.

2. Carbohydrate Management: Carbohydrates have the most significant impact on blood sugar levels. Choosing complex carbohydrates like whole grains, legumes, and vegetables, and being mindful of portion sizes, can help maintain steady blood sugar levels.

3. Protein for Muscle Maintenance: With age, maintaining muscle mass becomes essential. Including lean protein sources in your diet, such as fish, chicken, beans, and lentils, can help preserve muscle strength and manage blood sugar.

4. Healthy Fats: Incorporating healthy fats, like those found in avocados, nuts, and olive oil, can support heart health and provide sustained energy.

5. Fiber for Digestive Health: High-fiber foods, such as fruits, vegetables, and whole grains, not only help in blood sugar control but also aid in digestion, which can be a concern for many over 50.

6. Hydration: Adequate hydration is crucial, especially for those on certain diabetes medications that can increase the risk of dehydration.

Understanding these nutritional needs lays the foundation for making healthy food choices that support diabetes management and overall well-being in your later years.

Foods to Embrace and Avoid

In managing diabetes after 50, it's vital to know which foods can help stabilize blood sugar levels and which ones may cause harmful spikes. This knowledge allows for a more controlled and enjoyable diet.

Foods to Embrace:

1. Whole Grains: Foods like brown rice, quinoa, whole wheat bread, and oatmeal provide complex carbohydrates which are digested slower, helping to maintain steady blood sugar levels.

2. Lean Proteins: Incorporating lean meats, poultry, fish, tofu, and legumes can help maintain muscle mass and keep you feeling full, aiding in weight management.

3. Healthy Fats: Sources like avocados, nuts, seeds, and olive oil contribute to heart health and overall satiety without spiking blood sugar.

4. Fruits and Vegetables: A variety of colorful fruits and vegetables not only provide essential vitamins and minerals but also dietary fiber, which helps in blood sugar control. Opt for whole fruits rather than juices for added fiber.

5. Dairy or Alternatives: Low-fat dairy products or plant-based alternatives can provide calcium and protein. Look for unsweetened versions to avoid added sugars.

6. Herbs and Spices: They add flavor without extra calories or sodium. Some, like cinnamon, may even have blood sugar-lowering properties.

Foods to Avoid:

1. Refined Carbohydrates: White bread, pasta, and pastries can cause rapid blood sugar spikes and are low in nutritional value.

2. Sugary Snacks and Beverages: Foods and drinks high in added sugars, such as sodas, candies, and desserts, should be limited as they can lead to quick glucose increases.

3. High Sodium Foods: Excessive salt intake can contribute to hypertension, a common concern in diabetics over 50. Processed and canned foods often contain high sodium levels.

4. Saturated and Trans Fats: Found in fried foods, baked goods, and some animal products, these fats can worsen heart health, a critical aspect for diabetics.

5. Alcohol: If consumed, it should be in moderation, as it can affect blood sugar levels and interact with diabetes medications.

Understanding which foods to embrace and which to avoid is a key step in managing diabetes effectively, especially as you age. By making informed food choices, you can enjoy a diverse and nutritious diet that supports your health goals.

Reading Food Labels

Navigating food labels is an essential skill for managing diabetes, especially after 50. Understanding how to read and interpret these labels helps you make healthier choices and control your blood sugar levels. Here's a guide to the key components you should look for on food labels:

1. Serving Size and Servings Per Container: This is the basis for the rest of the information on the label. Note that the nutrient information provided is often for a single serving, not the entire package.

2. Total Carbohydrates: Pay close attention to this section. It includes sugars, complex carbohydrates, and fiber. For blood sugar management, look at the total carbohydrates rather than just the sugar content.

3. Fiber: High fiber content is beneficial for diabetes management as it slows down the absorption of sugars, helping to stabilize blood sugar levels. Aim for foods high in dietary fiber.

4. Sugars: This includes both added sugars and those naturally occurring in foods. Foods with low added sugars are preferable.

5. *Total Fat:* Look for foods low in saturated and trans fats. The type of fat is more important than the amount when it comes to diabetes and heart health.

6. *Protein:* A vital nutrient, especially for muscle maintenance in older adults. It also has a minimal impact on blood sugar levels.

7. *Sodium:* High sodium can be a concern for blood pressure, a common issue in diabetics. Opt for lower sodium options.

8. *Ingredients List:* Ingredients are listed in order of quantity. Look for whole food ingredients and be wary of items with long lists of unrecognizable ingredients.

9. *Nutrient Claims:* Be cautious of terms like "low-fat" or "sugar-free." Low-fat products might have added sugars, and sugar-free items might be high in carbohydrates or fats.

10. *Percent Daily Values (%DV):* These give you an idea of how much a nutrient in a serving of food contributes to a daily diet. Use it as a guide to understand if a product is high or low in a particular nutrient.

Learning to read and understand food labels empowers you to make informed decisions about the foods you eat. This skill is essential in managing diabetes, especially for those over 50, as it directly impacts your ability to maintain stable blood sugar levels and a healthy weight.

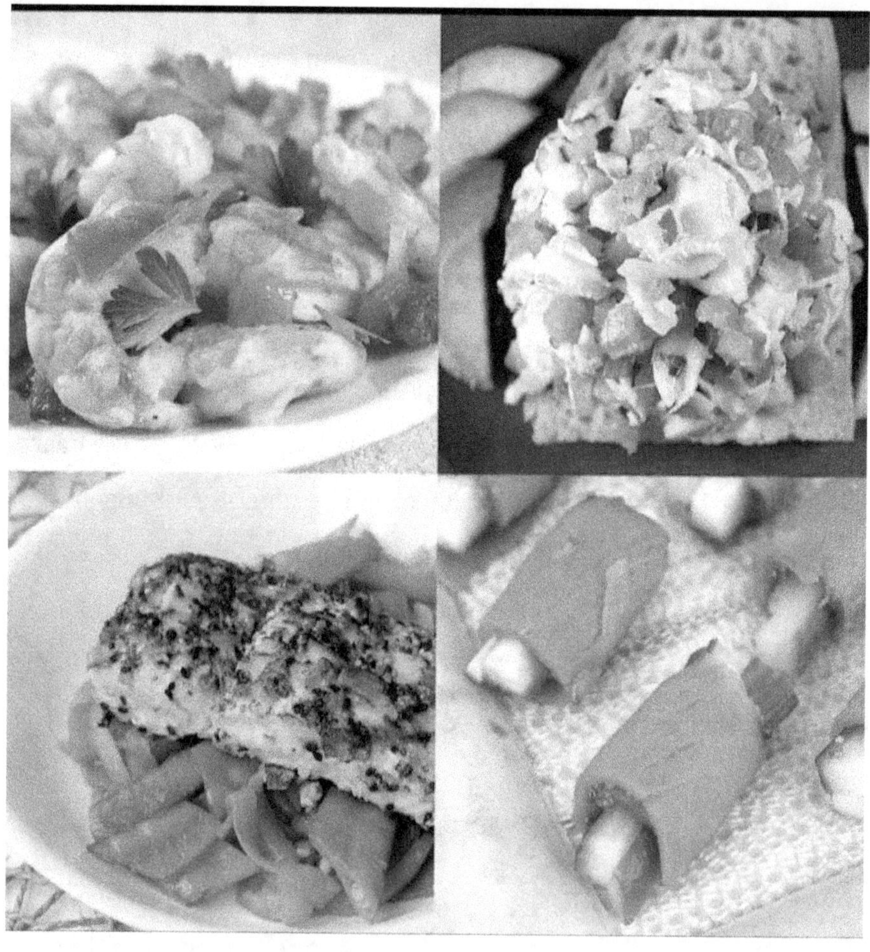

3. 50 DELICIOUS DIABETIC-FRIENDLY RECIPES

BREAKFASTS FOR A STRONG START

1. Almond and Blueberry Oatmeal

Prep Time: 5 minutes

Cook Time: 10 minutes

Serving Size: 1 bowl

Ingredients:

- ½ cup rolled oats

- 1 cup water or unsweetened almond milk

- ½ cup blueberries (fresh or frozen)

- 1 tablespoon chopped almonds

- 1 teaspoon honey (optional)

- ¼ teaspoon ground cinnamon

Nutritional Facts:

- Calories: 210 kcal

- Carbohydrates: 37 g

- Dietary Fiber: 6 g

- Sugars: 10 g

- Protein: 7 g

- Fat: 5 g

Preparation Directions:

1. In a small pot, combine the rolled oats and water (or almond milk). Bring to a boil, then reduce heat to simmer.
2. Cook for about 10 minutes, stirring occasionally, until the oats are soft and have absorbed the liquid.
3. Stir in the blueberries, almonds, honey (if using), and cinnamon.
4. Cook for an additional 2 minutes, then serve warm.

Health Benefit:

This oatmeal is ideal for diabetic patients over 50 due to its high fiber content, which helps in regulating blood sugar levels. The almonds add healthy fats and protein, aiding in prolonged energy and muscle maintenance.

2. Spinach and Feta Egg Muffins

Prep Time: 10 minutes
Cook Time: 20 minutes
Serving Size: 2 muffins

Ingredients:

- 4 large eggs
- 1 cup spinach, chopped
- ¼ cup feta cheese, crumbled

- ¼ cup red bell pepper, diced

- Salt and pepper to taste

- Cooking spray or olive oil

Nutritional Facts:

- Calories: 150 kcal (per 2 muffins)

- Carbohydrates: 2 g

- Dietary Fiber: 0.5 g

- Sugars: 1 g

- Protein: 12 g

- Fat: 10 g

Preparation Directions:

1. Preheat the oven to 350°F (175°C) and lightly grease a muffin pan with cooking spray or olive oil.

2. In a bowl, whisk together the eggs, salt, and pepper.

3. Add the chopped spinach, feta cheese, and diced bell pepper to the egg mixture.

4. Pour the mixture into the prepared muffin cups, filling each about ¾ full.

5. Bake for 20 minutes or until the muffins are set and lightly golden on top.

6. Allow to cool for a few minutes before serving.

Health Benefit:

These egg muffins are a protein-rich breakfast option, perfect for stabilizing blood sugar levels in the morning. The addition of spinach provides essential vitamins and minerals, supporting overall health for those over 50 with diabetes.

3. Greek Yogurt with Nuts and Berries

Prep Time: 5 minutes
Serving Size: 1 bowl

Ingredients:
- 1 cup Greek yogurt, unsweetened
- ½ cup mixed berries (strawberries, blueberries, raspberries)
- 2 tablespoons mixed nuts (almonds, walnuts, pecans), chopped
- 1 teaspoon honey (optional)

Nutritional Facts:
- Calories: 220 kcal
- Carbohydrates: 18 g
- Dietary Fiber: 3 g
- Sugars: 12 g
- Protein: 20 g
- Fat: 8 g

Preparation Directions:

1. In a serving bowl, add the Greek yogurt.

2. Top with mixed berries and chopped nuts.

3. Drizzle with honey if desired.

4. Mix gently and enjoy.

Health Benefit:

This recipe is an excellent source of high-quality protein from Greek yogurt, vital for muscle maintenance in older adults. The berries provide antioxidants and fiber, aiding in blood sugar regulation and overall heart health.

4. Avocado Toast on Whole Grain Bread

Prep Time: 5 minutes
Cook Time: 2 minutes
Serving Size: 1 slice

Ingredients:

- 1 slice whole grain bread

- ½ ripe avocado

- Salt and pepper to taste

- Red pepper flakes (optional)

Nutritional Facts:

- Calories: 180 kcal

- Carbohydrates: 20 g

- Dietary Fiber: 7 g

- Sugars: 3 g

- Protein: 6 g

- Fat: 10 g

Preparation Directions:

1. Toast the whole grain bread to your liking.

2. Mash the avocado and spread it evenly over the toast.

3. Season with salt, pepper, and red pepper flakes if desired.

Health Benefit:

Avocado toast offers a balance of healthy fats, fiber, and protein. The monounsaturated fats in avocado are beneficial for heart health, while the fiber from whole grain bread helps in maintaining steady blood sugar levels.

5. Cottage Cheese and Peach Bowl

Prep Time: 5 minutes

Serving Size: 1 bowl

Ingredients:

- 1 cup cottage cheese, low-fat

- 1 peach, sliced

- 1 tablespoon chopped walnuts

- 1 teaspoon honey (optional)

Nutritional Facts:

- Calories: 200 kcal

- Carbohydrates: 18 g

- Dietary Fiber: 2 g

- Sugars: 16 g

- Protein: 18 g

- Fat: 6 g

Preparation Directions:

1. In a serving bowl, add the cottage cheese.

2. Top with sliced peach and chopped walnuts.

3. Drizzle with honey if desired.

Health Benefit:

The combination of low-fat cottage cheese and peach makes for a protein-rich and low-glycemic breakfast. It's ideal for maintaining steady blood sugar levels, and the addition of walnuts provides healthy fats for heart health.

6. Veggie-Packed Breakfast Scramble

Prep Time: 5 minutes
Cook Time: 10 minutes
Serving Size: 1 serving

Ingredients:

- 2 large eggs

- ¼ cup bell peppers, diced

- ¼ cup onions, diced

- ¼ cup tomatoes, diced

- ¼ cup spinach, chopped

- 1 tablespoon olive oil

- Salt and pepper to taste

Nutritional Facts:

- Calories: 250 kcal

- Carbohydrates: 8 g

- Dietary Fiber: 2 g

- Sugars: 4 g

- Protein: 14 g

- Fat: 18 g

Preparation Directions:

1. Heat olive oil in a skillet over medium heat.
2. Add the diced bell peppers and onions, sautéing until they are soft.
3. Beat the eggs in a bowl and pour them into the skillet.
4. As the eggs begin to set, add the tomatoes and spinach.
5. Stir gently, cooking until the eggs are fully cooked.
6. Season with salt and pepper to taste, and serve hot.

Health Benefit:

This Veggie-Packed Breakfast Scramble is rich in nutrients and provides a balanced mix of protein, healthy fats, and fiber. The vegetables add essential vitamins and minerals, supporting overall health and aiding in blood sugar management for individuals over 50 with diabetes.

7. Chia Seed and Berry Parfait

Prep Time: 10 minutes (plus overnight soaking)
Serving Size: 1 parfait

Ingredients:

- 3 tablespoons chia seeds

- 1 cup unsweetened almond milk

- ½ cup mixed berries (strawberries, blueberries, raspberries)

- 1 tablespoon chopped nuts (optional)

- 1 teaspoon honey (optional)

Nutritional Facts:

- Calories: 220 kcal

- Carbohydrates: 24 g

- Dietary Fiber: 14 g

- Sugars: 6 g

- Protein: 8 g

- Fat: 12 g

Preparation Directions:

1. In a bowl, mix the chia seeds with almond milk. Stir well and let it sit overnight in the refrigerator.

2. The next morning, stir the chia seed mixture to ensure there are no clumps.

3. In a serving glass or bowl, layer the chia seed mixture with mixed berries.

4. Top with chopped nuts and a drizzle of honey if desired.

Health Benefit:

Chia seeds are a fantastic source of fiber, omega-3 fatty acids, and protein, making this parfait a nutrient-dense choice for managing diabetes. The high fiber content aids in blood sugar control, and the berries provide antioxidants without a significant sugar spike.

8. Whole Wheat Apple Pancakes

Prep Time: 10 minutes
Cook Time: 15 minutes
Serving Size: 2 pancakes

Ingredients:

- ½ cup whole wheat flour

- 1 medium apple, grated

- 1 large egg

- ½ cup unsweetened almond milk

- 1 teaspoon baking powder

- ½ teaspoon ground cinnamon

- 1 tablespoon olive oil (for cooking)

- Sugar-free maple syrup (optional for serving)

Nutritional Facts:

- Calories: 280 kcal

- Carbohydrates: 42 g

- Dietary Fiber: 6 g

- Sugars: 10 g

- Protein: 10 g

- Fat: 10 g

Preparation Directions:

1. In a mixing bowl, combine whole wheat flour, baking powder, and ground cinnamon.
2. Add the grated apple, egg, and almond milk to the dry ingredients. Mix until well combined.
3. Heat olive oil in a skillet over medium heat.
4. Pour batter to form pancakes in the skillet. Cook for about 2-3 minutes on each side or until golden brown.
5. Serve warm with sugar-free maple syrup if desired.

Health Benefit:

These Whole Wheat Apple Pancakes offer a hearty, fiber-rich breakfast option. The whole wheat flour and apple provide dietary fiber, aiding in blood sugar control and digestion. The added cinnamon not only enhances flavor but also has potential blood sugar regulating properties.

9. Turkey and Spinach Omelette

Prep Time: 5 minutes

Cook Time: 10 minutes

Serving Size: 1 omelette

Ingredients:

- 2 large eggs

- ¼ cup cooked turkey breast, chopped

- ¼ cup spinach, chopped

- 2 tablespoons feta cheese, crumbled

- 1 tablespoon olive oil

- Salt and pepper to taste

Nutritional Facts:

- Calories: 300 kcal

- Carbohydrates: 2 g

- Dietary Fiber: 0.5 g

- Sugars: 1 g

- Protein: 28 g

- Fat: 20 g

Preparation Directions:

1. Beat the eggs in a bowl and season with salt and pepper.

2. Heat olive oil in a skillet over medium heat.

3. Pour the eggs into the skillet, letting them spread to cover the base.

4. As the eggs begin to set, add the chopped turkey, spinach, and crumbled feta cheese.

5. Fold the omelette in half and cook until the eggs are fully set.

6. Serve hot, garnished with additional spinach if desired.

Health Benefit:

This protein-packed Turkey and Spinach Omelette is ideal for maintaining muscle mass and keeping blood sugar levels stable. The addition of spinach adds valuable nutrients like iron and folate, important for overall health in diabetics over 50.

10. Quinoa and Fruit Breakfast Bowl

Prep Time: 5 minutes (if using pre-cooked quinoa)
Cook Time: 20 minutes (for cooking quinoa)
Serving Size: 1 bowl

Ingredients:

- ½ cup cooked quinoa

- ½ banana, sliced

- ¼ cup blueberries

- 1 tablespoon chopped nuts

- 1 teaspoon honey (optional)

- A pinch of cinnamon

Nutritional Facts:

- Calories: 230 kcal

- Carbohydrates: 39 g

- Dietary Fiber: 5 g

- Sugars: 11 g

- Protein: 8 g

- Fat: 6 g

Preparation Directions:

1. If not using pre-cooked quinoa, cook quinoa according to package instructions and let it cool.
2. In a serving bowl, add the cooked quinoa.
3. Top with sliced banana, blueberries, and chopped nuts.
4. Drizzle with honey and sprinkle cinnamon on top.

Health Benefit:

Quinoa is a high-protein, gluten-free grain that makes an excellent base for a diabetic-friendly breakfast. It has a low glycemic index, ensuring a slow and steady release of glucose into the bloodstream. The fruits add natural sweetness and vitamins without significantly spiking blood sugar levels.

11. Grilled Chicken Salad with Mixed Greens

Prep Time: 15 minutes

Cook Time: 10 minutes

Serving Size: 1 salad

Ingredients:

- 1 boneless, skinless chicken breast

- 2 cups mixed greens (spinach, arugula, lettuce)

- ½ cup cherry tomatoes, halved

- ¼ cucumber, sliced

- 2 tablespoons balsamic vinaigrette

- 1 tablespoon olive oil

- Salt and pepper to taste

Nutritional Facts:

- Calories: 300 kcal

- Carbohydrates: 8 g

- Dietary Fiber: 3 g

- Sugars: 4 g

- Protein: 35 g

- Fat: 14 g

Preparation Directions:

1. Season the chicken breast with salt and pepper.

2. Grill the chicken over medium heat with olive oil until fully cooked and juicy, about 5 minutes per side.

3. Let the chicken rest for a few minutes, then slice it.

4. In a large bowl, mix the mixed greens, cherry tomatoes, and cucumber.

5. Add the sliced chicken on top of the greens.

6. Drizzle with balsamic vinaigrette and toss gently to combine.

Health Benefit:

This salad is a protein-rich, low-carb option perfect for a diabetic diet. The mixed greens provide essential vitamins and minerals, while the chicken offers lean protein that helps in blood sugar regulation and muscle maintenance.

12. Lentil Soup with Vegetables

Prep Time: 10 minutes

Cook Time: 30 minutes

Serving Size: 1 bowl

Ingredients:

- 1 cup lentils, rinsed

- 4 cups vegetable broth

- 1 carrot, diced

- 1 celery stalk, diced

- 1 onion, diced

- 2 garlic cloves, minced

- 1 teaspoon olive oil

- Salt and pepper to taste

- ½ teaspoon ground cumin

Nutritional Facts:

- Calories: 220 kcal

- Carbohydrates: 35 g

- Dietary Fiber: 15 g

- Sugars: 4 g

- Protein: 14 g

- Fat: 3 g

Preparation Directions:

1. In a large pot, heat the olive oil over medium heat.
2. Add the onion, carrot, celery, and garlic. Cook until the vegetables are softened.
3. Add the lentils, vegetable broth, cumin, salt, and pepper.
4. Bring to a boil, then reduce heat and simmer for about 30 minutes, or until the lentils are tender.
5. Adjust seasoning to taste and serve hot.

Health Benefit:

Lentils are an excellent source of fiber and protein, making this soup a great choice for blood sugar management. The high fiber content aids in slow digestion and provides a steady release of glucose, beneficial for diabetic patients over 50.

13. Turkey and Avocado Wrap

Prep Time: 10 minutes

Serving Size: 1 wrap

Ingredients:

- 1 whole grain tortilla wrap

- 2 slices of turkey breast

- ½ ripe avocado, sliced

- ¼ cup lettuce, shredded

- 2 tablespoons Greek yogurt

- 1 tablespoon mustard

- Salt and pepper to taste

Nutritional Facts:

- Calories: 320 kcal

- Carbohydrates: 30 g

- Dietary Fiber: 6 g

- Sugars: 4 g

- Protein: 22 g

- Fat: 14 g

Preparation Directions:

1. Lay the whole grain tortilla flat on a plate.

2. Spread Greek yogurt and mustard over the tortilla.

3. Place the turkey slices, avocado, and lettuce on top.

4. Season with salt and pepper.

5. Roll the tortilla tightly, then cut in half and serve.

Health Benefit:

This wrap combines lean protein from the turkey and healthy fats from the avocado, contributing to a balanced and heart-healthy meal. The whole grain tortilla adds fiber, which is key for controlling blood sugar levels.

14. Quinoa and Black Bean Salad

Prep Time: 15 minutes

Cook Time: 20 minutes (for quinoa)

Serving Size: 1 serving

Ingredients:

- ½ cup cooked quinoa

- ½ cup black beans, drained and rinsed

- ½ red bell pepper, diced

- 2 tablespoons red onion, finely chopped

- 2 tablespoons cilantro, chopped

- 1 tablespoon lime juice

- 1 tablespoon olive oil

- Salt and pepper to taste

Nutritional Facts:

- Calories: 330 kcal

- Carbohydrates: 45 g

- Dietary Fiber: 10 g

- Sugars: 3 g

- Protein: 12 g

- Fat: 13 g

Preparation Directions:

1. In a bowl, combine cooked quinoa, black beans, red bell pepper, red onion, and cilantro.
2. In a small bowl, whisk together lime juice, olive oil, salt, and pepper.
3. Pour the dressing over the quinoa mixture and toss to combine.
4. Serve chilled or at room temperature.

Health Benefit:

This salad is rich in plant-based protein and fiber, making it an excellent choice for diabetic patients over 50. The combination of quinoa and black beans provides a complete protein, while the fiber helps in maintaining stable blood sugar levels.

15. Tuna Salad Stuffed Bell Peppers

Prep Time: 15 minutes

Serving Size: 1 stuffed pepper

Ingredients:

- 1 large bell pepper, halved and seeded
- 1 can (5 oz) tuna in water, drained
- 2 tablespoons mayonnaise, light
- 1 tablespoon celery, finely chopped
- 1 tablespoon red onion, finely chopped

- 1 teaspoon lemon juice

- Salt and pepper to taste

- Fresh parsley for garnish (optional)

Nutritional Facts:

- Calories: 190 kcal (per half)

- Carbohydrates: 8 g

- Dietary Fiber: 2 g

- Sugars: 4 g

- Protein: 22 g

- Fat: 8 g

Preparation Directions:

1. In a bowl, mix the tuna, mayonnaise, celery, red onion, lemon juice, salt, and pepper.
2. Fill each bell pepper half with the tuna salad mixture.
3. Garnish with fresh parsley if desired.
4. Serve chilled.

Health Benefit:

Tuna is a great source of lean protein and omega-3 fatty acids, beneficial for heart health and blood sugar control. The bell peppers provide a low-carb alternative to bread, rich in vitamins and antioxidants.

16. Cauliflower Rice Stir-Fry

Prep Time: 10 minutes

Cook Time: 15 minutes

Serving Size: 1 serving

Ingredients:

- 1 cup cauliflower rice

- ½ cup mixed vegetables (carrots, peas, bell peppers)

- 1 egg, beaten

- 1 garlic clove, minced

- 2 tablespoons soy sauce, low sodium

- 1 tablespoon olive oil

- Salt and pepper to taste

Nutritional Facts:

- Calories: 180 kcal

- Carbohydrates: 15 g

- Dietary Fiber: 4 g

- Sugars: 5 g

- Protein: 9 g

- Fat: 10 g

Preparation Directions:

1. Heat olive oil in a skillet over medium heat.

2. Add garlic and sauté until fragrant.

3. Add the mixed vegetables and cook until they are soft.

4. Stir in the cauliflower rice and cook for 5 minutes.

5. Push the cauliflower rice to one side of the skillet and add the beaten egg to the other side.

6. Scramble the egg and then mix it with the cauliflower rice.

7. Add soy sauce, salt, and pepper, and stir well to combine.

8. Serve hot.

Health Benefit:

Cauliflower rice provides a low-carb, high-fiber alternative to traditional rice, making it an excellent choice for blood sugar management. The vegetables add vitamins and minerals, while the egg provides a good source of protein.

17. Spinach and Mushroom Frittata

Prep Time: 10 minutes

Cook Time: 20 minutes

Serving Size: 1 slice

Ingredients:

- 4 large eggs

- 1 cup spinach, chopped

- ½ cup mushrooms, sliced

- ¼ cup onions, diced

- 2 tablespoons Parmesan cheese, grated

- 1 tablespoon olive oil

- Salt and pepper to taste

Nutritional Facts:

- Calories: 160 kcal (per slice)

- Carbohydrates: 3 g

- Dietary Fiber: 1 g

- Sugars: 2 g

- Protein: 12 g

- Fat: 11 g

Preparation Directions:

1. Preheat the oven to 350°F (175°C).

2. Heat olive oil in an oven-safe skillet over medium heat.

3. Sauté onions, mushrooms, and spinach until the spinach is wilted.

4. In a bowl, whisk together eggs, Parmesan cheese, salt, and pepper.

5. Pour the egg mixture over the vegetables in the skillet.

6. Cook for 3-4 minutes until the edges begin to set.

7. Transfer the skillet to the oven and bake for 15 minutes or until the frittata is set.

8. Serve warm.

Health Benefit:

This frittata is a protein-rich and low-carb meal, making it suitable for blood sugar management. The spinach and mushrooms provide essential nutrients and antioxidants, supporting overall health in diabetic patients over 50.

18. Baked Sweet Potato with Cottage Cheese

Prep Time: 5 minutes

Cook Time: 45 minutes

Serving Size: 1 serving

Ingredients:

- 1 medium sweet potato

- ½ cup cottage cheese, low-fat

- 1 tablespoon chives, chopped

- Salt and pepper to taste

Nutritional Facts:

- Calories: 220 kcal

- Carbohydrates: 35 g

- Dietary Fiber: 5 g

- Sugars: 12 g

- Protein: 15 g

- Fat: 2 g

Preparation Directions:

1. Preheat the oven to 400°F (200°C).
2. Pierce the sweet potato with a fork and place it on a baking sheet.
3. Bake for 45 minutes, or until tender.
4. Split the sweet potato open and fluff the inside with a fork.
5. Top with cottage cheese and chives.
6. Season with salt and pepper to taste.

Health Benefit:

Sweet potatoes are a great source of complex carbohydrates and fiber. Paired with protein-rich cottage cheese, this meal provides sustained energy and aids in blood sugar stability, beneficial for diabetic patients over 50.

19. Chickpea and Cucumber Salad

Prep Time: 10 minutes

Serving Size: 1 serving

Ingredients:

- 1 cup chickpeas, drained and rinsed

- 1 cucumber, diced

- ½ red onion, finely chopped

- 2 tablespoons parsley, chopped

- 2 tablespoons lemon juice

- 1 tablespoon olive oil

- Salt and pepper to taste

Nutritional Facts:

- Calories: 250 kcal

- Carbohydrates: 35 g

- Dietary Fiber: 10 g

- Sugars: 7 g

- Protein: 10 g

- Fat: 8 g

Preparation Directions:

1. In a large bowl, combine chickpeas, cucumber, red onion, and parsley.
2. In a small bowl, whisk together lemon juice, olive oil, salt, and pepper.
3. Pour the dressing over the salad and toss to combine.
4. Serve chilled or at room temperature.

Health Benefit:

This salad is rich in plant-based protein and fiber from the chickpeas, making it an excellent choice for blood sugar control. The cucumber and parsley provide hydration and essential vitamins, supporting overall health.

20. Broccoli and Chicken Casserole

Prep Time: 15 minutes

Cook Time: 30 minutes

Serving Size: 1 serving

Ingredients:

- 1 cup broccoli florets

- 1 boneless, skinless chicken breast, cooked and shredded

- ½ cup Greek yogurt, plain

- ¼ cup cheddar cheese, shredded

- 1 garlic clove, minced

- 1 tablespoon olive oil

- Salt and pepper to taste

Nutritional Facts:

- Calories: 350 kcal

- Carbohydrates: 10 g

- Dietary Fiber: 3 g

- Sugars: 4 g

- Protein: 40 g

- Fat: 16 g

Preparation Directions:

1. Preheat the oven to 375°F (190°C).

2. Steam the broccoli until just tender, about 3-4 minutes.

3. In a mixing bowl, combine the shredded chicken, Greek yogurt, half of the cheese, garlic, salt, and pepper.

4. Stir in the steamed broccoli.

5. Transfer the mixture to a baking dish and sprinkle the remaining cheese on top.

6. Bake for 25-30 minutes, or until the cheese is melted and bubbly.

7. Serve hot.

Health Benefit:

This casserole combines lean protein from the chicken and nutrient-rich broccoli, making it an ideal meal for blood sugar management. The Greek yogurt provides a creamy texture without the excess fat, supporting heart health.

21. Salmon with Steamed Asparagus

Prep Time: 10 minutes
Cook Time: 15 minutes
Serving Size: 1 serving

Ingredients:

- 1 salmon fillet (6 oz)

- 1 cup asparagus spears

- 1 tablespoon olive oil

- 1 lemon, zest and juice

- Salt and pepper to taste

- Dill for garnish (optional)

Nutritional Facts:

- Calories: 370 kcal

- Carbohydrates: 5 g

- Dietary Fiber: 2 g

- Sugars: 2 g

- Protein: 34 g

- Fat: 24 g

Preparation Directions:

1. Preheat the oven to 400°F (200°C).

2. Season the salmon with salt, pepper, and lemon zest.

3. Place the salmon on a baking sheet lined with parchment paper.

4. Drizzle olive oil and lemon juice over the salmon.

5. Arrange asparagus around the salmon.

6. Bake for 12-15 minutes or until the salmon is cooked through and asparagus is tender.

7. Garnish with dill before serving.

Health Benefit:

Salmon is rich in omega-3 fatty acids, crucial for heart health and managing inflammation, making it an excellent choice for diabetic patients over 50. Asparagus is a low-carb vegetable high in vitamins and fiber, supporting blood sugar control.

22. Grilled Vegetable and Tofu Skewers

Prep Time: 15 minutes (plus marinating time)
Cook Time: 10 minutes
Serving Size: 2 skewers

Ingredients:

- 1 block firm tofu, cut into cubes

- 1 zucchini, sliced

- 1 red bell pepper, cut into pieces

- 1 onion, cut into wedges

- 2 tablespoons soy sauce, low sodium

- 1 tablespoon olive oil

- 1 garlic clove, minced

- Salt and pepper to taste

Nutritional Facts:

- Calories: 250 kcal

- Carbohydrates: 15 g

- Dietary Fiber: 4 g

- Sugars: 6 g

- Protein: 16 g

- Fat: 14 g

Preparation Directions:

1. In a bowl, mix soy sauce, olive oil, garlic, salt, and pepper
    for the marinade.

2. Add tofu cubes to the marinade and let sit for at least 30
    minutes.

3. Preheat the grill to medium-high heat.

4. Thread tofu and vegetables alternately onto skewers.

5. Grill for 10 minutes, turning occasionally, until vegetables
    are tender and tofu is slightly charred.

6. Serve hot.

Health Benefit:

These skewers are a plant-based meal rich in protein and fiber.
Tofu is a low-fat protein source, and the vegetables provide
essential nutrients and antioxidants, supporting overall health in
diabetic patients.

23. Beef and Broccoli Stir-Fry

Prep Time: 10 minutes

Cook Time: 15 minutes

Serving Size: 1 serving

Ingredients:

- 4 oz lean beef, sliced thinly

- 1 cup broccoli florets

- 1 garlic clove, minced

- 1 tablespoon soy sauce, low sodium

- 1 teaspoon sesame oil

- 1 teaspoon ginger, grated

- ½ tablespoon cornstarch

- ½ cup water or beef broth, low sodium

- Salt and pepper to taste

- 1 tablespoon olive oil

Nutritional Facts:

- Calories: 280 kcal

- Carbohydrates: 12 g

- Dietary Fiber: 3 g

- Sugars: 2 g

- Protein: 27 g

- Fat: 15 g

Preparation Directions:

1. In a bowl, mix cornstarch, soy sauce, sesame oil, ginger, and water/beef broth to make the sauce.
2. Heat olive oil in a skillet over medium-high heat.
3. Add beef and stir-fry until browned. Remove beef and set aside.
4. In the same skillet, add garlic and broccoli. Stir-fry until the broccoli is tender.
5. Return the beef to the skillet and pour the sauce over it.
6. Cook until the sauce thickens and coats the beef and broccoli.
7. Season with salt and pepper, and serve.

Health Benefit:

Lean beef is an excellent source of protein and iron, essential for muscle maintenance and energy levels. Broccoli, being high in fiber and vitamins, aids in digestion and provides antioxidants beneficial for overall health.

24. Baked Eggplant Parmesan

Prep Time: 15 minutes

Cook Time: 30 minutes

Serving Size: 1 serving

Ingredients:

- 1 medium eggplant, sliced

- 1 cup marinara sauce, low sodium

- ½ cup mozzarella cheese, part-skim, shredded

- 2 tablespoons Parmesan cheese, grated

- 1 teaspoon olive oil

- 1 garlic clove, minced

- Salt and pepper to taste

- Fresh basil for garnish

Nutritional Facts:

- Calories: 320 kcal

- Carbohydrates: 35 g

- Dietary Fiber: 8 g

- Sugars: 15 g

- Protein: 18 g

- Fat: 15 g

Preparation Directions:

1. Preheat the oven to 375°F (190°C).
2. Brush eggplant slices with olive oil and season with salt, pepper, and minced garlic.
3. Bake eggplant slices for 15 minutes, turning once until they are slightly browned.
4. In a baking dish, layer eggplant, marinara sauce, and cheeses.
5. Repeat the layers and finish with cheese on top.
6. Bake for an additional 15 minutes or until the cheese is melted and bubbly.
7. Garnish with fresh basil and serve hot.

Health Benefit:

Eggplant is a low-carb, high-fiber vegetable making it ideal for blood sugar management. The cheeses provide calcium and protein, essential for bone health and muscle maintenance in older adults.

25. Zucchini Noodles with Pesto Chicken

Prep Time: 20 minutes
Cook Time: 20 minutes
Serving Size: 1 serving

Ingredients:

- 1 large zucchini, spiralized

- 1 chicken breast, grilled and sliced

- 2 tablespoons pesto sauce

- 1 tablespoon olive oil

- Salt and pepper to taste

- Parmesan cheese for garnish (optional)

Nutritional Facts:

- Calories: 400 kcal

- Carbohydrates: 8 g

- Dietary Fiber: 2 g

- Sugars: 4 g

- Protein: 36 g

- Fat: 24 g

Preparation Directions:

1. Spiralize the zucchini into noodles.
2. In a skillet, heat olive oil over medium heat.
3. Add zucchini noodles and sauté for 3-5 minutes until tender.
4. Add the grilled chicken slices and pesto sauce. Toss to combine.
5. Cook for an additional 2-3 minutes.
6. Season with salt and pepper, and garnish with Parmesan cheese if desired.

Health Benefit:

Zucchini noodles provide a low-carb, high-fiber alternative to traditional pasta, beneficial for blood sugar control. Chicken is a lean protein source, and the pesto adds healthy fats, making this a balanced meal for diabetic patients over 50.

26. Shrimp and Cauliflower Grits

Prep Time: 15 minutes

Cook Time: 20 minutes

Serving Size: 1 serving

Ingredients:

- ½ lb shrimp, peeled and deveined

- 2 cups cauliflower, riced

- 1 cup chicken broth, low sodium

- 2 tablespoons cream cheese, low-fat

- 1 garlic clove, minced

- 1 tablespoon olive oil

- Salt and pepper to taste

- Paprika and parsley for garnish

Nutritional Facts:

- Calories: 320 kcal

- Carbohydrates: 15 g

- Dietary Fiber: 4 g

- Sugars: 5 g

- Protein: 35 g

- Fat: 14 g

Preparation Directions:

1. In a skillet, heat olive oil over medium heat.

2. Add garlic and shrimp, season with salt, pepper, and paprika. Cook until shrimp are pink and set aside.

3. In a saucepan, bring chicken broth to a boil. Add riced cauliflower and cook until tender.

4. Stir in cream cheese until the mixture reaches a creamy consistency.

5. Serve the shrimp over cauliflower grits.

6. Garnish with parsley.

Health Benefit:

Shrimp is a great source of lean protein, while cauliflower provides a low-carb, high-fiber alternative to traditional grits. This combination aids in blood sugar control and supports heart health, beneficial for diabetic patients over 50.

27. Turkey Meatballs with Spaghetti Squash

Prep Time: 20 minutes
Cook Time: 40 minutes
Serving Size: 1 serving

Ingredients:

- 1 spaghetti squash, halved and seeds removed

- ½ lb ground turkey

- 1 egg

- ¼ cup breadcrumbs, whole wheat

- 1 garlic clove, minced

- 1 teaspoon Italian seasoning

- 1 cup marinara sauce, low sodium

- Salt and pepper to taste

- Olive oil

Nutritional Facts:

- Calories: 450 kcal

- Carbohydrates: 40 g

- Dietary Fiber: 8 g

- Sugars: 12 g

- Protein: 35 g

- Fat: 18 g

Preparation Directions:

1. Preheat the oven to 400°F (200°C).
2. Brush the inside of the spaghetti squash with olive oil and season with salt and pepper. Place cut side down on a baking sheet and bake for 40 minutes.
3. In a bowl, combine ground turkey, egg, breadcrumbs, garlic, Italian seasoning, salt, and pepper. Form into meatballs.
4. In a skillet, cook the meatballs until browned on all sides.
5. Pour marinara sauce over the meatballs and simmer until cooked through.
6. Use a fork to shred the cooked spaghetti squash into strands.
7. Serve the meatballs over the spaghetti squash.

Health Benefit:

This dish provides a low-carb alternative to traditional pasta dishes. Spaghetti squash is high in fiber and vitamins, and ground turkey offers lean protein, making it a hearty yet healthy choice for managing diabetes.

28. Stuffed Bell Peppers with Ground Turkey

Prep Time: 20 minutes
Cook Time: 30 minutes
Serving Size: 1 pepper

Ingredients:

- 2 bell peppers, halved and seeded

- ½ lb ground turkey

- 1 cup quinoa, cooked

- 1 onion, diced

- 1 garlic clove, minced

- 1 cup tomato sauce, low sodium

- ¼ cup cheese, part-skim mozzarella, shredded

- 1 tablespoon olive oil

- Salt and pepper to taste

- Italian seasoning

Nutritional Facts:

- Calories: 350 kcal (per stuffed pepper)

- Carbohydrates: 30 g

- Dietary Fiber: 5 g

- Sugars: 8 g

- Protein: 25 g

- Fat: 15 g

Preparation Directions:

1. Preheat the oven to 375°F (190°C).

2. In a skillet, heat olive oil and cook the onion, garlic, and ground turkey. Season with salt, pepper, and Italian seasoning.

3. Mix in cooked quinoa and tomato sauce.

4. Fill each bell pepper half with the turkey and quinoa mixture.

5. Top with shredded cheese.

6. Bake for 30 minutes or until the peppers are tender.

7. Serve hot.

Health Benefit:

Bell peppers are rich in vitamins and low in carbohydrates, making them an excellent choice for a diabetic-friendly meal. Combined with protein-rich ground turkey and fiber-filled quinoa, this dish supports balanced blood sugar levels.

29. Vegetable and Lentil Stew

Prep Time: 15 minutes

Cook Time: 45 minutes

Serving Size: 1 bowl

Ingredients:

- 1 cup lentils, rinsed

- 4 cups vegetable broth

- 1 carrot, diced

- 1 potato, diced

- 1 onion, diced

- 2 garlic cloves, minced

- 1 can diced tomatoes

- 1 teaspoon olive oil

- Salt and pepper to taste

- Italian seasoning

Nutritional Facts:

- Calories: 280 kcal

- Carbohydrates: 45 g

- Dietary Fiber: 15 g

- Sugars: 8 g

- Protein: 14 g

- Fat: 4 g

Preparation Directions:

1. In a large pot, heat olive oil over medium heat.
2. Add onions, garlic, carrots, and potatoes. Cook until vegetables are soft.
3. Add lentils, diced tomatoes, vegetable broth, Italian seasoning, salt, and pepper.
4. Bring to a boil, then reduce heat and simmer for 45 minutes or until lentils are tender.
5. Adjust seasoning to taste and serve hot.

Health Benefit:

Lentils are a great source of plant-based protein and fiber, which are key for blood sugar management. The vegetables add essential nutrients and antioxidants, supporting overall health in diabetic patients.

30. Baked Lemon Garlic Tilapia

Prep Time: 10 minutes

Cook Time: 15 minutes

Serving Size: 1 fillet

Ingredients:

- 1 tilapia fillet (6 oz)

- 1 lemon, juice and zest

- 1 garlic clove, minced

- 1 tablespoon olive oil

- Salt and pepper to taste

- Parsley for garnish

Nutritional Facts:

- Calories: 220 kcal

- Carbohydrates: 3 g

- Dietary Fiber: 1 g

- Sugars: 1 g

- Protein: 34 g

- Fat: 9 g

Preparation Directions:

1. Preheat the oven to 400°F (200°C).
2. In a small bowl, mix together lemon juice and zest, minced garlic, olive oil, salt, and pepper.
3. Place the tilapia fillet on a baking sheet lined with parchment paper.
4. Pour the lemon garlic mixture over the tilapia.
5. Bake for 12-15 minutes or until the fish flakes easily with a fork.
6. Garnish with parsley before serving.

Health Benefit:

Tilapia is a lean source of protein, essential for muscle maintenance. The lemon and garlic not only add flavor but also provide vitamin C and anti-inflammatory benefits, making this dish a light yet nutritious option for dinner.

HEALTHY SNACKS AND SIDES

31. Carrot and Hummus Dip

Prep Time: 10 minutes
Serving Size: 1 serving

Ingredients:

- 1 large carrot, peeled and sliced

- ¼ cup hummus

Nutritional Facts:

- Calories: 120 kcal

- Carbohydrates: 16 g

- Dietary Fiber: 5 g

- Sugars: 5 g

- Protein: 4 g

- Fat: 5 g

Preparation Directions:

1. Simply peel and slice the carrot into sticks.

2. Serve with a side of hummus for dipping.

Health Benefit:

Carrots are a great source of beta-carotene and fiber, while hummus provides protein and healthy fats. This snack is ideal for blood sugar management, making it perfect for diabetic patients over 50.

32. Greek Yogurt and Mixed Nuts

Prep Time: 5 minutes

Serving Size: 1 bowl

Ingredients:

- 1 cup Greek yogurt, unsweetened

- ¼ cup mixed nuts (almonds, walnuts, pecans)

Nutritional Facts:

- Calories: 280 kcal

- Carbohydrates: 10 g

- Dietary Fiber: 2 g

- Sugars: 7 g

- Protein: 25 g

- Fat: 16 g

Preparation Directions:

1. Scoop the Greek yogurt into a bowl.

2. Top with a mixture of nuts.

Health Benefit:

Greek yogurt is high in protein and calcium, essential for bone health and muscle maintenance. The nuts provide healthy fats and additional protein, making this a satisfying snack that supports blood sugar control.

33. Apple Slices with Almond Butter

Prep Time: 5 minutes

Serving Size: 1 serving

Ingredients:

- 1 apple, sliced

- 2 tablespoons almond butter

Nutritional Facts:

- Calories: 180 kcal

- Carbohydrates: 25 g

- Dietary Fiber: 5 g

- Sugars: 17 g

- Protein: 4 g

- Fat: 9 g

Preparation Directions:

1. Slice the apple.

2. Serve with almond butter for dipping.

Health Benefit:

Apples provide fiber and essential vitamins, while almond butter offers healthy fats and protein. This combination makes for a balanced snack, aiding in blood sugar stability and satiety.

34. Cottage Cheese with Pineapple

Prep Time: 5 minutes
Serving Size: 1 bowl

Ingredients:

- 1 cup cottage cheese, low-fat
- ½ cup pineapple, diced

Nutritional Facts:

- Calories: 200 kcal

- Carbohydrates: 20 g

- Dietary Fiber: 1 g

- Sugars: 15 g

- Protein: 22 g

- Fat: 3 g

Preparation Directions:

1. Combine the cottage cheese and diced pineapple in a bowl.

Health Benefit:

Cottage cheese is an excellent source of protein and calcium, while pineapple provides vitamin C and a hint of natural sweetness. This snack is great for muscle maintenance and offers a refreshing taste.

35. Baked Kale Chips

Prep Time: 10 minutes

Cook Time: 15 minutes

Serving Size: 1 cup

Ingredients:

- 2 cups kale leaves, washed and torn

- 1 tablespoon olive oil

- Salt and pepper to taste

Nutritional Facts:

- Calories: 80 kcal

- Carbohydrates: 7 g

- Dietary Fiber: 2 g

- Sugars: 0 g

- Protein: 3 g

- Fat: 5 g

Preparation Directions:

1. Preheat the oven to 350°F (175°C).

2. Toss kale leaves with olive oil, salt, and pepper.

3. Spread the leaves on a baking sheet in a single layer.

4. Bake for 10-15 minutes or until crisp.

5. Let them cool before serving.

Health Benefit:

Kale chips are a low-calorie, nutrient-dense snack rich in vitamins A, C, and K. They provide a crunchy satisfaction without the high carbs of traditional chips, making them ideal for blood sugar control.

36. Roasted Chickpeas

Prep Time: 5 minutes
Cook Time: 30 minutes
Serving Size: 1 cup

Ingredients:

- 1 can (15 oz) chickpeas, drained and rinsed

- 1 tablespoon olive oil

- Salt and pepper to taste

- Your choice of seasonings (e.g., paprika, garlic powder, cumin)

Nutritional Facts:

- Calories: 210 kcal

- Carbohydrates: 35 g

- Dietary Fiber: 10 g

- Sugars: 6 g

- Protein: 10 g

- Fat: 4 g

Preparation Directions:

1. Preheat the oven to 400°F (200°C).
2. Pat the chickpeas dry and toss them with olive oil, salt, pepper, and your chosen seasonings.
3. Spread the chickpeas on a baking sheet in a single layer.
4. Roast for 25-30 minutes, stirring halfway through, until crispy.
5. Let them cool before serving.

Health Benefit:

Roasted chickpeas are a high-fiber, high-protein snack, making them great for blood sugar control. They provide a crunchy texture and can be seasoned in various ways for a tasty treat.

37. Mixed Berry Fruit Salad

Prep Time: 10 minutes

Serving Size: 1 cup

Ingredients:

- ¼ cup strawberries, sliced

- ¼ cup blueberries

- ¼ cup raspberries

- ¼ cup blackberries

- 1 tablespoon lemon juice

- 1 teaspoon honey (optional)

Nutritional Facts:

- Calories: 70 kcal

- Carbohydrates: 17 g

- Dietary Fiber: 5 g

- Sugars: 10 g

- Protein: 1 g

- Fat: 0.5 g

Preparation Directions:

1. Combine all the berries in a bowl.

2. Drizzle with lemon juice and honey if desired.

3. Toss gently to combine and serve.

Health Benefit:

Berries are packed with antioxidants and are low in sugar compared to other fruits, making them a great choice for diabetic patients. They also provide essential vitamins and fiber, aiding in overall health and blood sugar management.

38. Celery Sticks with Peanut Butter

Prep Time: 5 minutes

Serving Size: 2 sticks

Ingredients:

- 2 celery sticks

- 2 tablespoons peanut butter, unsweetened

Nutritional Facts:

- Calories: 190 kcal

- Carbohydrates: 8 g

- Dietary Fiber: 3 g

- Sugars: 4 g

- Protein: 8 g

- Fat: 15 g

Preparation Directions:

1. Wash and cut the celery sticks to your preferred size.

2. Spread peanut butter evenly on each celery stick.

Health Benefit:

Celery is low in calories and provides a satisfying crunch, while peanut butter offers healthy fats and protein. This snack helps in maintaining steady blood sugar levels and provides lasting energy.

39. Sliced Cucumber and Cream Cheese

Prep Time: 5 minutes

Serving Size: 1 serving

Ingredients:

- 1 medium cucumber, sliced
- ¼ cup cream cheese, low-fat

Nutritional Facts:

- Calories: 100 kcal
- Carbohydrates: 6 g
- Dietary Fiber: 1 g
- Sugars: 3 g
- Protein: 3 g
- Fat: 7 g

Preparation Directions:

1. Slice the cucumber into rounds.

2. Spread a small amount of cream cheese on each cucumber slice.

Health Benefit:

This snack is refreshing and light, with the cucumber providing hydration and the cream cheese offering a source of protein and calcium. It's a balanced snack that's easy on blood sugar levels.

40. Roasted Almonds and Walnuts

Prep Time: 5 minutes

Cook Time: 10 minutes

Serving Size: ¼ cup

Ingredients:

- ½ cup almonds

- ½ cup walnuts

- Salt to taste (optional)

Nutritional Facts:

- Calories: 200 kcal

- Carbohydrates: 6 g

- Dietary Fiber: 3 g

- Sugars: 1 g

- Protein: 5 g

- Fat: 18 g

Preparation Directions:

1. Preheat the oven to 350°F (175°C).

2. Spread almonds and walnuts on a baking sheet in a single layer.

3. Roast for 10 minutes, stirring occasionally.

4. Season with a pinch of salt if desired.

Health Benefit:

Nuts are a great source of healthy fats, protein, and fiber, making them an ideal snack for blood sugar management. They are heart-healthy and can help keep you full and satisfied between meals.

DESSERTS AND SWEET TREATS

41. Baked Apple with Cinnamon

Prep Time: 5 minutes

Cook Time: 30 minutes

Serving Size: 1 apple

Ingredients:

- 1 large apple, cored

- ½ teaspoon cinnamon

- 1 tablespoon chopped walnuts

- 1 teaspoon honey (optional)

Nutritional Facts:

- Calories: 120 kcal

- Carbohydrates: 25 g

- Dietary Fiber: 5 g

- Sugars: 18 g

- Protein: 1 g

- Fat: 3 g

Preparation Directions:

1. Preheat the oven to 350°F (175°C).
2. Place the cored apple on a baking dish.
3. Mix cinnamon and walnuts together, then stuff into the apple core.
4. Drizzle with honey if desired.
5. Bake for 30 minutes or until the apple is tender.
6. Serve warm.

Health Benefit:

Baked apple with cinnamon is a sweet treat that's naturally low in calories and high in fiber. The cinnamon adds flavor without sugar, making it a good choice for blood sugar management.

42. Dark Chocolate and Almond Clusters

Prep Time: 10 minutes

Cook Time: 0 minutes (chill time 30 minutes)

Serving Size: 2 clusters

Ingredients:

- ½ cup dark chocolate chips, at least 70% cocoa

- ¼ cup almonds, whole or sliced

Nutritional Facts:

- Calories: 150 kcal

- Carbohydrates: 12 g

- Dietary Fiber: 2 g

- Sugars: 8 g

- Protein: 3 g

- Fat: 10 g

Preparation Directions:

1. Melt dark chocolate chips in a microwave-safe bowl in 30-second intervals, stirring until smooth.

2. Mix almonds into the melted chocolate.

3. Spoon small clusters of the mixture onto a parchment-lined tray.

4. Chill in the refrigerator for 30 minutes or until set.

5. Serve cold.

Health Benefit:

Dark chocolate is rich in antioxidants and almonds provide healthy fats and protein. This dessert is a satisfying treat that's heart-healthy and diabetic-friendly.

43. Strawberry and Chia Pudding

Prep Time: 10 minutes (plus overnight soaking)

Serving Size: 1 cup

Ingredients:

- 2 tablespoons chia seeds

- ½ cup unsweetened almond milk

- ½ cup strawberries, chopped

- 1 teaspoon honey (optional)

Nutritional Facts:

- Calories: 150 kcal

- Carbohydrates: 18 g

- Dietary Fiber: 10 g

- Sugars: 6 g

- Protein: 5 g

- Fat: 7 g

Preparation Directions:

1. In a bowl, mix chia seeds with almond milk. Let it sit overnight in the refrigerator.
2. Stir the mixture to break any clumps.
3. Top with chopped strawberries and a drizzle of honey if desired.
4. Serve cold.

Health Benefit:

Chia seeds are high in fiber and omega-3 fatty acids, making this pudding a great choice for maintaining blood sugar levels and heart health. Strawberries add natural sweetness and vitamin C.

44. Peach and Cottage Cheese Crepes

Prep Time: 20 minutes

Cook Time: 10 minutes

Serving Size: 2 crepes

Ingredients:

- 2 crepes (whole wheat or low-carb)

- ½ cup cottage cheese, low-fat

- 1 peach, sliced

- 1 teaspoon honey (optional)

- Cinnamon to taste

Nutritional Facts:

- Calories: 220 kcal

- Carbohydrates: 30 g

- Dietary Fiber: 3 g

- Sugars: 16 g

- Protein: 12 g

- Fat: 5 g

Preparation Directions:

1. Lay out the crepes on a flat surface.

2. Spread cottage cheese over each crepe.

3. Arrange peach slices on top of the cottage cheese.

4. Drizzle with honey and sprinkle with cinnamon if desired.

5. Roll up the crepes and serve.

Health Benefit:

Peach and cottage cheese crepes provide a balanced combination of protein, healthy carbs, and fiber. Cottage cheese is high in protein, while peaches offer natural sweetness and fiber, aiding in blood sugar control.

45. Raspberry Coconut Milk Smoothie

Prep Time: 5 minutes

Serving Size: 1 smoothie

Ingredients:

- 1 cup raspberries, fresh or frozen

- ½ cup coconut milk, unsweetened

- ½ banana, optional for sweetness

- 1 tablespoon chia seeds

- 1 teaspoon honey (optional)

- Ice cubes (optional)

Nutritional Facts:

- Calories: 180 kcal

- Carbohydrates: 20 g

- Dietary Fiber: 8 g

- Sugars: 9 g (without banana)

- Protein: 3 g

- Fat: 10 g

Preparation Directions:

1. In a blender, combine raspberries, coconut milk, banana (if using), chia seeds, and honey.

2. Add ice cubes if you prefer a colder smoothie.

3. Blend until smooth and creamy.

4. Pour into a glass and serve immediately.

Health Benefit:

This smoothie is rich in antioxidants from the raspberries and healthy fats from the coconut milk. Chia seeds add fiber and omega-3 fatty acids, making it a nutritious and satisfying treat that can help manage blood sugar levels for diabetic patients over 50.

46. Lemon Ricotta Berry Cups

Prep Time: 10 minutes
Serving Size: 1 cup

Ingredients:

- ½ cup ricotta cheese, low-fat

- 1 tablespoon lemon zest

- ½ cup mixed berries (blueberries, raspberries, strawberries)

- 1 teaspoon honey (optional)

- Mint leaves for garnish (optional)

Nutritional Facts:

- Calories: 150 kcal

- Carbohydrates: 12 g

- Dietary Fiber: 2 g

- Sugars: 8 g

- Protein: 10 g

- Fat: 7 g

Preparation Directions:

1. In a bowl, mix the ricotta cheese with lemon zest.

2. Spoon the ricotta mixture into a serving cup.

3. Top with mixed berries.

4. Drizzle with honey and garnish with mint leaves if desired.

Health Benefit:

Lemon Ricotta Berry Cups offer a high-protein, low-carb dessert option. The ricotta provides calcium and protein, while the berries add antioxidants and fiber, making it a balanced treat for blood sugar control.

47. Baked Pear with Honey and Walnuts

Prep Time: 5 minutes
Cook Time: 30 minutes
Serving Size: 1 serving

Ingredients:

- 1 pear, halved and cored

- 1 tablespoon honey

- 2 tablespoons walnuts, chopped

- Cinnamon to taste

Nutritional Facts:

- Calories: 200 kcal

- Carbohydrates: 35 g

- Dietary Fiber: 6 g

- Sugars: 27 g

- Protein: 2 g

- Fat: 7 g

Preparation Directions:

1. Preheat the oven to 350°F (175°C).

2. Place pear halves on a baking dish, cut side up.

3. Drizzle with honey and sprinkle with cinnamon.

4. Top with chopped walnuts.

5. Bake for 30 minutes or until the pear is tender.

6. Serve warm.

Health Benefit:

Pears are a fiber-rich fruit, beneficial for digestion and blood sugar control. Combined with walnuts, which provide healthy fats and protein, this dessert is both nutritious and satisfying.

48. Chocolate Avocado Mousse

Prep Time: 10 minutes

Serving Size: 1 cup

Ingredients:

- 1 ripe avocado

- 2 tablespoons cocoa powder, unsweetened

- 2 tablespoons honey or maple syrup

- ½ teaspoon vanilla extract

- A pinch of salt

Nutritional Facts:

- Calories: 250 kcal

- Carbohydrates: 30 g

- Dietary Fiber: 7 g

- Sugars: 20 g

- Protein: 4 g

- Fat: 15 g

Preparation Directions:

1. Scoop the avocado flesh into a blender.

2. Add cocoa powder, honey/maple syrup, vanilla extract, and salt.

3. Blend until smooth and creamy.

4. Refrigerate for 30 minutes before serving.

Health Benefit:

This mousse provides healthy fats from the avocado and antioxidants from the cocoa. It's a dairy-free, low-carb dessert, making it an excellent choice for managing blood sugar levels while satisfying sweet cravings.

49. Almond Flour Blueberry Muffins

Prep Time: 15 minutes

Cook Time: 20 minutes

Serving Size: 1 muffin

Ingredients:

- 1½ cups almond flour

- ½ cup blueberries

- 2 eggs

- ¼ cup honey or maple syrup

- 1 teaspoon baking powder

- 1 teaspoon vanilla extract

- A pinch of salt

Nutritional Facts:

- Calories: 150 kcal (per muffin)

- Carbohydrates: 10 g

- Dietary Fiber: 2 g

- Sugars: 6 g

- Protein: 5 g

- Fat: 11 g

Preparation Directions:

1. Preheat the oven to 350°F (175°C) and line a muffin tin with paper liners.
2. In a bowl, mix almond flour, baking powder, and salt.
3. In another bowl, whisk together eggs, honey, and vanilla extract.
4. Combine wet and dry ingredients. Gently fold in blueberries.
5. Fill muffin cups and bake for 20 minutes or until a toothpick inserted comes out clean.
6. Let cool before serving.

Health Benefit:

Almond flour muffins are a low-carb alternative to traditional muffins, making them suitable for blood sugar management. Blue berries add natural sweetness and antioxidants.

50. Grilled Peaches with Greek Yogurt

Prep Time: 5 minutes
Cook Time: 10 minutes
Serving Size: 1 serving

Ingredients:

- 1 peach, halved and pitted

- ½ cup Greek yogurt, unsweetened

- 1 teaspoon honey (optional)

- Cinnamon to taste

Nutritional Facts:

- Calories: 120 kcal

- Carbohydrates: 18 g

- Dietary Fiber: 2 g

- Sugars: 16 g

- Protein: 10 g

- Fat: 0.5 g

Preparation Directions:

1. Preheat a grill or grill pan over medium heat.
2. Place peach halves cut side down on the grill. Cook for 5 minutes or until grill marks appear.
3. Flip and cook for another 5 minutes.
4. Serve warm with a dollop of Greek yogurt on each half.
5. Drizzle with honey and sprinkle with cinnamon.

Health Benefit:

Grilled peaches provide a sweet, low-calorie dessert option. Paired with Greek yogurt, this dish offers protein and probiotics, aiding digestion and overall health, beneficial for diabetic patients.

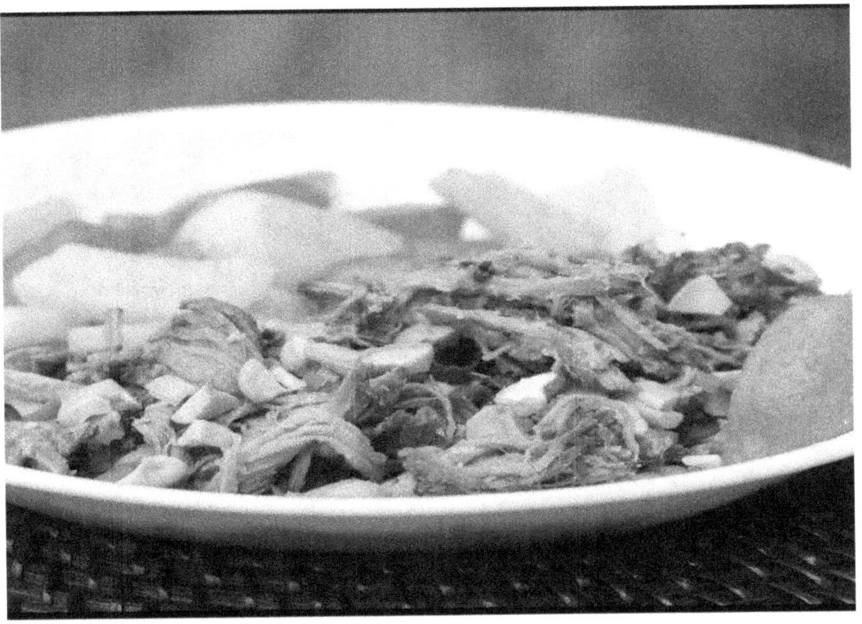

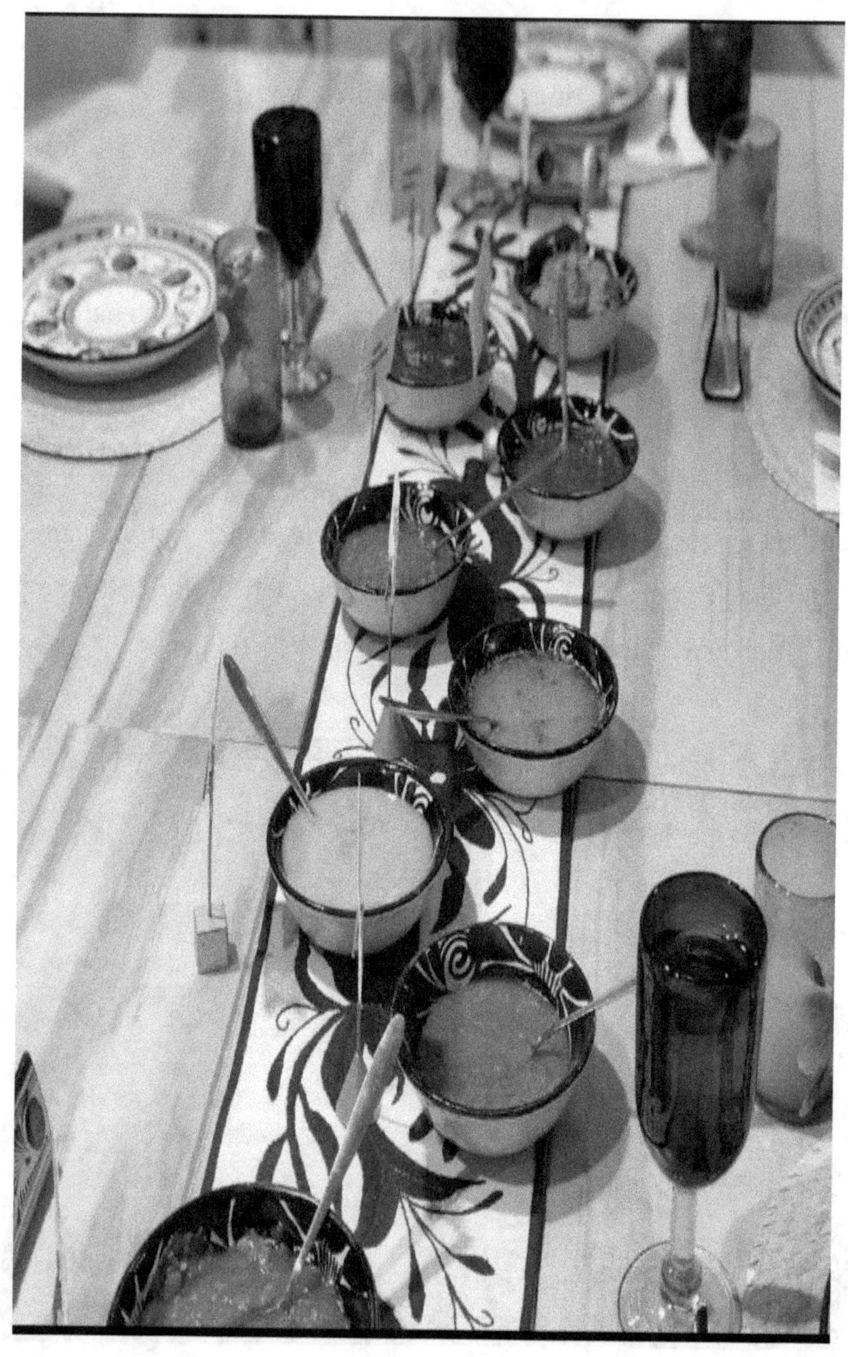

4. SPECIAL DIETARY CONSIDERATION

Managing diabetes effectively after the age of 50 often requires paying attention to other health concerns as well. This section of "Diabetic Diets Cookbook After 50" focuses on special dietary considerations to address various health needs. Each subsection provides guidance and tailored recipes to help you maintain a balanced and healthy diet while managing diabetes and other health conditions.

Heart-Healthy Options

Eating for heart health is crucial, especially for those managing diabetes. Diabetes can increase the risk of heart disease, making it essential to incorporate heart-healthy foods into your diet.

Key Considerations for Heart-Healthy Eating:
- **Opt for Healthy Fats:** Focus on unsaturated fats found in foods like avocados, nuts, seeds, and olive oil. These fats can help lower cholesterol levels.

- **Increase Fiber Intake:** High-fiber foods like whole grains, fruits, and vegetables can help lower blood cholesterol and improve heart health.

- **Limit Saturated and Trans Fats:** Reduce intake of high-fat meats, full-fat dairy products, and processed foods to keep cholesterol in check.

- **Incorporate Omega-3 Fatty Acids:** Foods rich in omega-3s, such as salmon, mackerel, and flaxseeds, are beneficial for heart health.

- **Control Portion Sizes:** Eating in moderation is key to maintaining a healthy weight and reducing strain on the heart.

Sample Heart-Healthy Recipes:

1. **Grilled Salmon with Quinoa and Spinach Salad:** A dish rich in omega-3 fatty acids and fiber.

2. **Avocado and Walnut Salad:** Offers a good mix of healthy fats and antioxidants.

3. **Oatmeal with Berries and Flaxseeds:** A breakfast option high in fiber and omega-3s.

4. **Vegetable Stir-Fry with Tofu:** Provides unsaturated fats and a variety of nutrients from vegetables.

5. **Chicken and Vegetable Soup with Whole Grain Bread:** A comforting meal high in protein and fiber, low in saturated fat.

Eating for heart health involves choosing foods that support cardiovascular function while also managing blood sugar levels. The recipes and tips in this section are designed to help you enjoy a diverse and flavorful diet that benefits your heart.

Low Sodium Choices

For diabetic patients over 50, managing sodium intake is crucial, particularly for those with high blood pressure or a risk of heart disease. Consuming too much sodium can lead to hypertension, a common condition in diabetics, which increases the risk of cardiovascular problems.

Key Strategies for Low Sodium Eating:

- **Choose Fresh Foods:** Fresh fruits, vegetables, and unprocessed meats are naturally low in sodium.

- **Read Labels Carefully:** Processed and packaged foods often contain high levels of sodium. Look for products labeled "low sodium" or "no salt added."

- **Cook at Home:** Preparing meals at home allows you to control the amount of salt added.

- **Use Herbs and Spices:** Enhance flavors with herbs, spices, garlic, vinegar, and lemon juice instead of salt.

- **Avoid High-Sodium Foods:** Limit or avoid foods like cured meats, canned soups, and fast foods.

Sample Low Sodium Recipes:

1. **Herb-Roasted Chicken with Vegetables:** A flavorful dish using herbs and spices instead of salt.

2. **Quinoa Salad with Fresh Vegetables and Lemon Dressing:** A refreshing, nutrient-rich meal with natural flavors.

3. **Homemade Vegetable Soup:** Control the salt content by making your own broth and using fresh ingredients.

4. **Grilled Fish with Mango Salsa:** A tasty way to enjoy seafood without added sodium.

5. **Stir-Fried Tofu and Broccoli in Garlic Sauce:** Use low-sodium soy sauce and plenty of garlic for flavor.

Adopting a low sodium diet can significantly improve heart health and blood pressure control. The recipes in this section are designed to be delicious and satisfying, helping you manage your sodium intake without sacrificing taste.

Gluten-Free Alternatives

Adopting a gluten-free diet can be essential for individuals with celiac disease or gluten sensitivity, and it can also be a choice for those looking for alternative grains and ingredients. For diabetic patients over 50, finding gluten-free options that are also diabetes-friendly is crucial to manage both blood sugar levels and digestive health.

Key Points for Gluten-Free Eating:

- **Understand Gluten Sources:** Gluten is found in wheat, barley, and rye. It's important to recognize these in ingredients lists.

- **Choose Naturally Gluten-Free Grains:** Quinoa, rice, buckwheat, and millet are great alternatives.

- **Read Labels for Hidden Gluten:** Gluten can be hidden in sauces, condiments, and processed foods. Always check labels.

- **Beware of Cross-Contamination:** Especially important for those with celiac disease, as even small amounts of gluten can cause issues.

- **Focus on Whole Foods:** Fruits, vegetables, meats, and dairy are naturally gluten-free and should form the basis of your diet.

Sample Gluten-Free Recipes:

1. **Quinoa and Black Bean Stuffed Peppers:** A filling meal packed with protein and fiber.

2. **Chicken and Vegetable Stir-Fry with Rice Noodles:** Use tamari sauce instead of soy sauce to keep it gluten-free.

3. **Buckwheat Pancakes with Berries:** Buckwheat is a nutritious, gluten-free alternative for breakfast.

4. **Rice Pilaf with Vegetables:** A versatile side dish that complements any meal.

5. **Almond Flour Blueberry Muffins:** A delicious, gluten-free snack that satisfies sweet cravings without spiking blood sugar.

Embracing gluten-free alternatives can lead to discovering a wide range of nutritious and tasty options that support both diabetes management and gluten sensitivity.

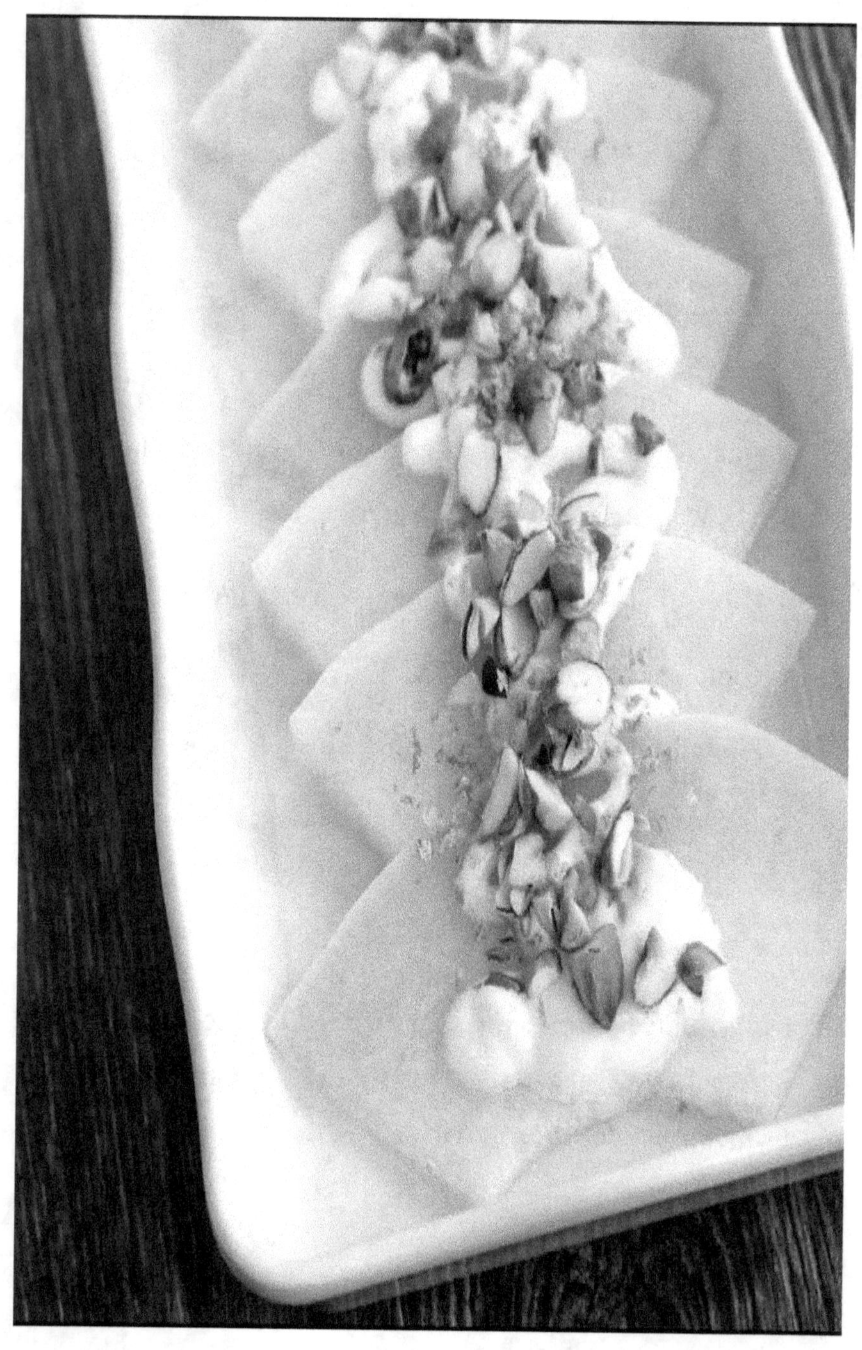

5. 14-DAY DIABETIC MEAL PLAN

Day 1

- Breakfast: Greek Yogurt with Nuts and Berries (#3)

- Lunch: Quinoa and Black Bean Salad (#14)

- Snack: Apple Slices with Almond Butter (#33)

- Dinner: Zucchini Noodles with Pesto Chicken (#25)

- Dessert: Dark Chocolate and Almond Clusters (#42)

Day 2

- Breakfast: Whole Wheat Apple Pancakes (#8)

- Lunch: Turkey and Avocado Wrap (#13)

- Snack: Carrot and Hummus Dip (#31)

- Dinner: Grilled Vegetable and Tofu Skewers (#22)

- Dessert: Raspberry Coconut Milk Smoothie (#45)

Day 3

- Breakfast: Veggie-Packed Breakfast Scramble (#6)

- Lunch: Lentil Soup with Vegetables (#12)

- Snack: Greek Yogurt and Mixed Nuts (#32)

- Dinner: Shrimp and Cauliflower Grits (#26)

- Dessert: Baked Apple with Cinnamon (#41)

Day 4

- Breakfast: Chia Seed and Berry Parfait (#7)

- Lunch: Spinach and Mushroom Frittata (#17)

- Snack: Roasted Chickpeas (#36)

- Dinner: Beef and Broccoli Stir-Fry (#23)

- Dessert: Strawberry and Chia Pudding (#43)

Day 5

- Breakfast: Avocado Toast on Whole Grain Bread (#4)

- Lunch: Cauliflower Rice Stir-Fry (#16)

- Snack: Sliced Cucumber and Cream Cheese (#39)

- Dinner: Baked Lemon Garlic Tilapia (#30)

- Dessert: Peach and Cottage Cheese Crepes (#44)

Day 6

- Breakfast: Almond and Blueberry Oatmeal (#1)

- Lunch: Grilled Chicken Salad with Mixed Greens (#11)

- Snack: Baked Kale Chips (#35)

- Dinner: Salmon with Steamed Asparagus (#21)

- Dessert: Lemon Ricotta Berry Cups (#46)

Day 7

- Breakfast: Turkey and Spinach Omelette (#9)

- Lunch: Broccoli and Chicken Casserole (#20)

- Snack: Mixed Berry Fruit Salad (#37)

- Dinner: Stuffed Bell Peppers with Ground Turkey (#28)

- Dessert: Baked Pear with Honey and Walnuts (#47)

Day 8

- Breakfast: Quinoa and Fruit Breakfast Bowl (#10)

- Lunch: Tuna Salad Stuffed Bell Peppers (#15)

- Snack: Roasted Almonds and Walnuts (#40)

- Dinner: Vegetable and Lentil Stew (#29)

- Dessert: Chocolate Avocado Mousse (#48)

Day 9

- Breakfast: Cottage Cheese and Peach Bowl (#5)

- Lunch: Grilled Chicken Salad with Mixed Greens (#11)

- Snack: Celery Sticks with Peanut Butter (#38)

- Dinner: Turkey Meatballs with Spaghetti Squash (#27)

- Dessert: Almond Flour Blueberry Muffins (#49)

Day 10

- Breakfast: Spinach and Feta Egg Muffins (#2)

- Lunch: Quinoa and Black Bean Salad (#14)

- Snack: Apple Slices with Almond Butter (#33)

- Dinner: Baked Eggplant Parmesan (#24)

- Dessert: Grilled Peaches with Greek Yogurt (#50)

Day 11

- Breakfast: Whole Wheat Apple Pancakes (#8)

- Lunch: Lentil Soup with Vegetables (#12)

- Snack: Greek Yogurt and Mixed Nuts (#32)

- Dinner: Zucchini Noodles with Pesto Chicken (#25)

- Dessert: Dark Chocolate and Almond Clusters (#42)

Day 12

- Breakfast: Veggie-Packed Breakfast Scramble (#6)

- Lunch: Turkey and Avocado Wrap (#13)

- Snack: Carrot and Hummus Dip (#31)

- Dinner: Shrimp and Cauliflower Grits (#26)

- Dessert: Raspberry Coconut Milk Smoothie (#45)

Day 13

- Breakfast: Chia Seed and Berry Parfait (#7)

- Lunch: Spinach and Mushroom Frittata (#17)

- Snack: Roasted Chickpeas (#36)

- Dinner: Beef and Broccoli Stir-Fry (#23)

- Dessert: Baked Apple with Cinnamon (#41)

Day 14

- Breakfast: Avocado Toast on Whole Grain Bread (#4)

- Lunch: Cauliflower Rice Stir-Fry (#16)

- Snack: Sliced Cucumber and Cream Cheese (#39)

- Dinner: Baked Lemon Garlic Tilapia (#30)

- Dessert: Peach and Cottage Cheese Crepes (#44)

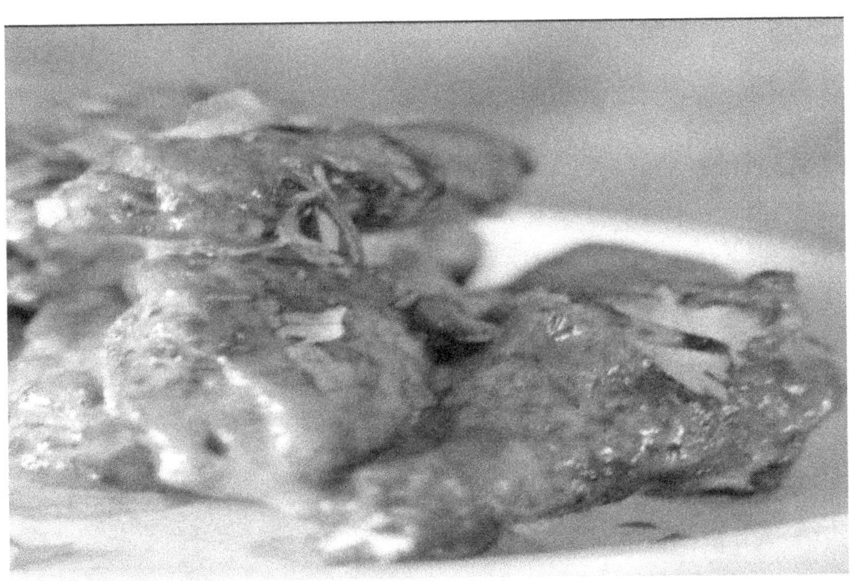

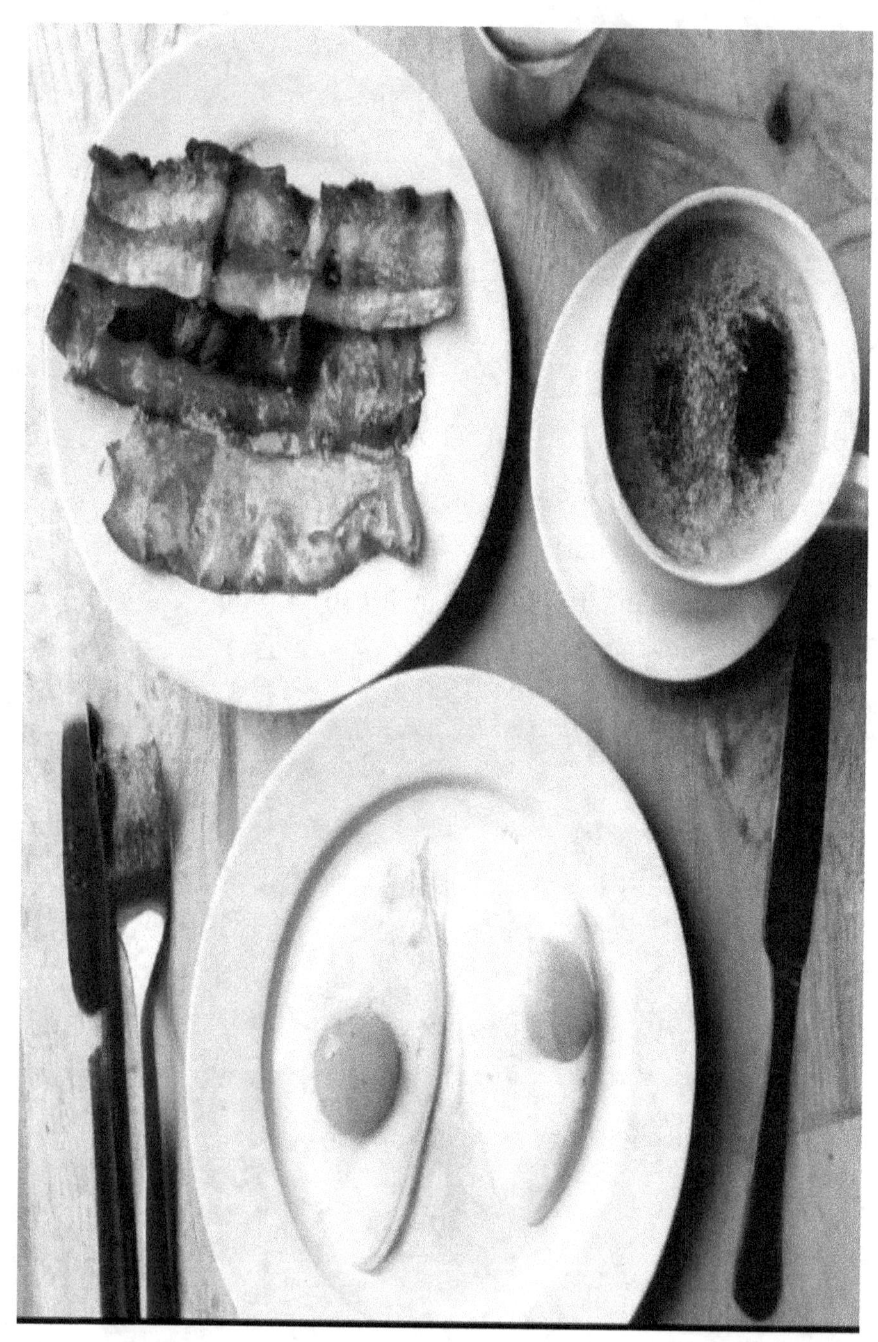

6. LIFESTYLE TIPS FOR MANAGING DIABETES AFTER 50

This section offers practical lifestyle tips for those over 50 managing diabetes. It's about more than just diet; it's about embracing a lifestyle that supports your overall health and well-being.

Exercise and Physical Activity

Regular exercise and physical activity are essential components of diabetes management, especially after the age of 50. Staying active helps control blood sugar levels, maintain a healthy weight, reduce the risk of heart disease, and improve overall mental health.

Key Tips for Incorporating Exercise:

- **Start Slowly:** If you're new to exercise, start with light activities like walking or gentle stretching. Gradually increase intensity and duration.

- **Aim for a Mix of Activities:** Include aerobic exercises (like walking, swimming, or cycling), strength training (using weights or resistance bands), and flexibility exercises (like yoga or tai chi).

- **Stay Consistent:** Aim for at least 150 minutes of moderate aerobic activity per week, as recommended by health experts.

- **Monitor Blood Sugar Levels:** Check your blood sugar before and after exercise, especially if you're taking insulin or medications that can cause low blood sugar.

- **Stay Hydrated and Be Prepared:** Carry a small carbohydrate snack in case your blood sugar levels drop during exercise.

- **Consult with Your Doctor:** Before starting any new exercise regimen, consult your healthcare provider, especially if you have any diabetes-related complications.

Regular physical activity not only helps in managing diabetes but also enhances your quality of life as you age. It can be a source of enjoyment and a way to connect with others too.

Stress Management Techniques

Managing stress is crucial for individuals over 50 with diabetes, as stress can significantly impact blood sugar levels and overall health. High stress levels can lead to poor blood sugar control, unhealthy eating habits, and a reduction in physical activity.

Effective Strategies for Stress Management:

- **Practice Mindfulness and Relaxation Techniques:** Activities like meditation, deep breathing exercises, and yoga can reduce stress and improve mental well-being.

- **Regular Physical Activity:** Exercise is not only good for your physical health but also for your mental health. It releases endorphins, natural stress relievers.

- **Maintain a Support Network:** Stay connected with friends, family, or support groups. Sharing your concerns and experiences with others can be therapeutic.

- **Establish a Routine:** A consistent daily routine can reduce stress by adding predictability to your day.

- **Get Adequate Sleep:** Poor sleep can exacerbate stress. Aim for 7-8 hours of quality sleep each night.

- **Engage in Hobbies:** Activities you enjoy can be great stress relievers. Whether it's gardening, reading, or crafting, hobbies can divert your mind from daily stressors.

- **Seek Professional Help if Needed:** If stress becomes overwhelming, consider speaking with a counselor or therapist specializing in stress management.

Implementing these stress management techniques can not only improve your ability to manage diabetes but also enhance your overall quality of life. Remember, taking care of your mental health is as important as taking care of your physical health.

Regular Health Check-Ups

Regular health check-ups are vital for managing diabetes effectively, especially for individuals over 50. As you age, your body undergoes various changes, and staying on top of your health becomes increasingly important. Regular monitoring and medical check-ups can help in early detection and management of potential complications associated with diabetes.

Key Aspects of Regular Health Check-Ups:

- **Consistent Blood Sugar Monitoring:** Regularly checking your blood sugar levels helps in making informed decisions about diet, exercise, and medication.

- **Routine A1C Testing:** This test measures your average blood sugar levels over the past 2-3 months and should be done at least twice a year.

- **Blood Pressure and Cholesterol Checks:** High blood pressure and cholesterol are common in people with diabetes and can increase the risk of heart disease and stroke.

- **Regular Eye Exams:** Diabetes can lead to eye problems like diabetic retinopathy. Annual eye exams are essential for early detection and treatment.

- **Kidney Function Tests:** Diabetes can affect kidney health. Regular urine and blood tests can assess how well your kidneys are functioning.

- **Foot Exams:** Diabetes can lead to nerve damage in the feet, so regular foot examinations are important to prevent infections and other complications.

- **Dental Check-Ups:** Diabetes increases the risk of gum disease, making regular dental visits important.

- **Vaccinations:** Stay up to date with vaccinations, as diabetes can weaken the immune system.

Communication with Healthcare Providers:

- **Keep Regular Appointments:** Even if you feel fine, it's important to see your healthcare provider regularly.

- **Be Open and Honest:** Share any concerns or symptoms you're experiencing with your healthcare team.

- **Discuss Medication Adjustments:** As your body changes, so may your medication needs. Regular discussions with your healthcare provider are key.

By prioritizing regular health check-ups and maintaining open communication with your healthcare team, you can manage diabetes more effectively and reduce the risk of complications as you age.

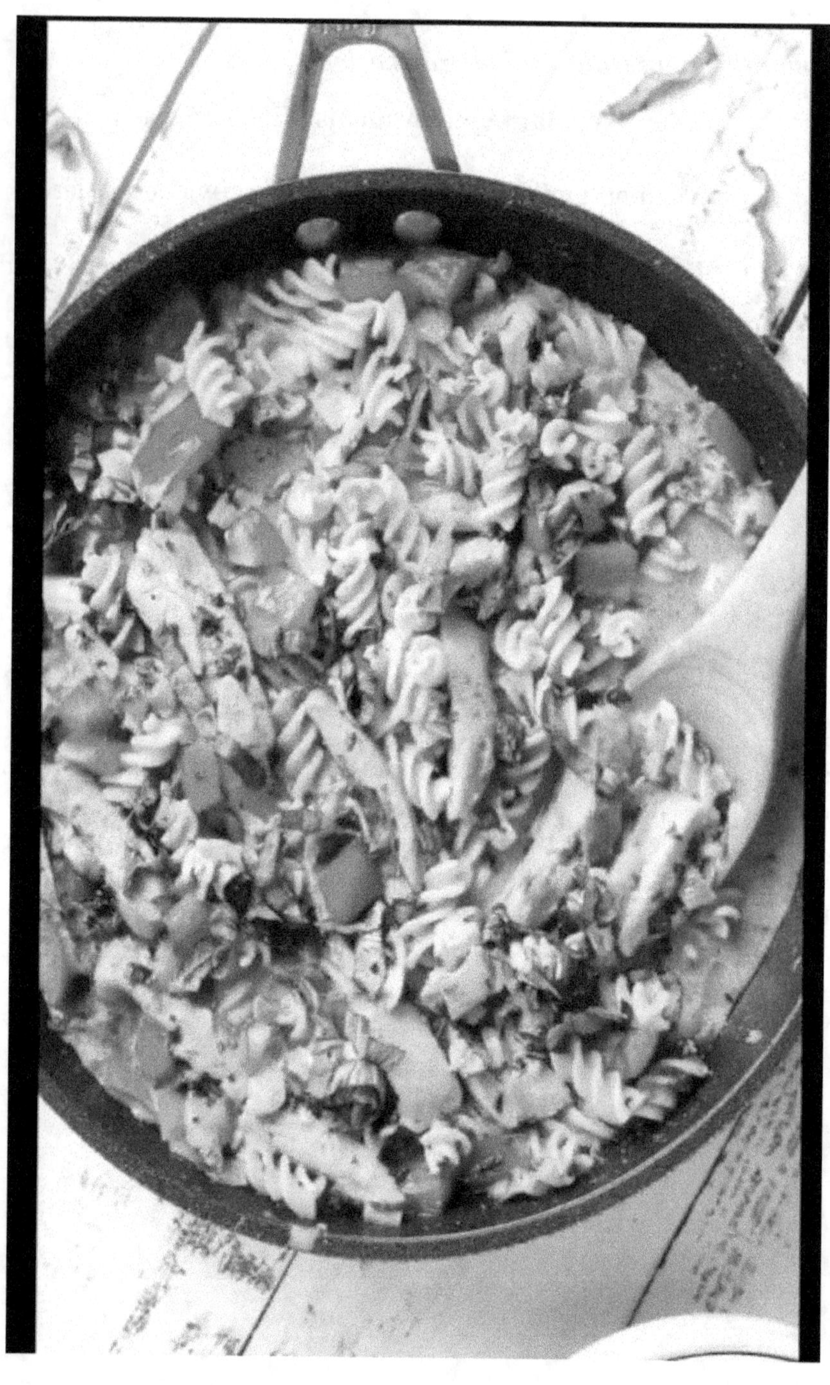

7. SHOPPING GUIDE AND BUDGET TIPS

Effective management of diabetes after 50 involves smart grocery shopping and budgeting. This section provides guidance on making informed choices while shopping and tips for keeping your grocery bills within budget.

Shopping List Essentials

Creating a shopping list is an essential tool for anyone managing diabetes. A well-thought-out list ensures you have all the necessary ingredients for your diabetic-friendly meals and helps you avoid impulse buys that might not align with your dietary goals.

Essential Categories and Items:

- **Fresh Produce:** Stock up on a variety of fruits and vegetables. Focus on leafy greens, berries, and non-starchy vegetables like broccoli, cauliflower, and bell peppers.

- **Whole Grains:** Choose whole grain or whole wheat options for bread, pasta, and rice. Look for high-fiber cereals and oats.

- **Lean Proteins:** Include sources like chicken breast, turkey, fish, eggs, and plant-based proteins like tofu and legumes.

- **Dairy or Alternatives:** Opt for low-fat or fat-free dairy products. For those who are lactose intolerant or vegan, almond milk, soy milk, and coconut yogurt are good alternatives.

- **Healthy Fats:** Avocados, nuts, seeds, and olive oil are excellent for heart health and overall well-being.

- **Frozen Produce:** Frozen fruits and vegetables can be a budget-friendly and convenient option. They are often frozen at peak freshness, retaining their nutrients.

- **Spices and Herbs:** Stock up on a variety of spices and herbs to add flavor to your meals without extra salt or sugar.

This shopping list focuses on nutrient-dense, whole foods that are beneficial for managing blood sugar levels and overall health for those over 50 with diabetes.

Budget-Friendly Shopping Tips

Eating healthily for diabetes management doesn't have to break the bank. There are several strategies to eat well while sticking to a budget. These tips can help you make the most of your grocery shopping, ensuring you get the best nutritional bang for your buck.

Effective Strategies for Budget-Conscious Shopping:

- **Plan Your Meals:** Create a meal plan for the week. This helps in buying only what you need, reducing waste and saving money.

- **Buy in Bulk:** Purchase non-perishable items or freezable foods in bulk. Items like whole grains, nuts, and frozen vegetables are often cheaper in larger quantities.

- **Shop Seasonal Produce:** Fruits and vegetables are less expensive when they are in season. Plus, they're at their peak flavor and nutritional value.

- **Use Coupons and Check Deals:** Look for coupons, sales, and promotions in grocery stores. Many stores offer discounts on certain items weekly.

- **Compare Prices:** Look at the unit price on shelf tags to compare different brands and sizes.

- **Consider Store Brands:** Store-brand products are often similar in quality to name brands but are less expensive.

- **Buy Frozen or Canned:** Frozen and canned fruits and vegetables (without added sugars or sodium) are good alternatives to fresh produce and often cheaper.

- **Limit Processed Foods:** Not only are they generally less healthy, but processed foods are often more expensive than whole foods.

- **Cook at Home:** Preparing meals at home is usually more economical than eating out. Plus, it's easier to manage your diet.

- **Use Leftovers Wisely:** Get creative with leftovers to make new meals, reducing food waste and saving money.

Implementing these tips can make a significant difference in your grocery bills. Eating healthily on a budget requires a bit of planning and smart shopping, but it's certainly achievable and beneficial for managing diabetes after 50.

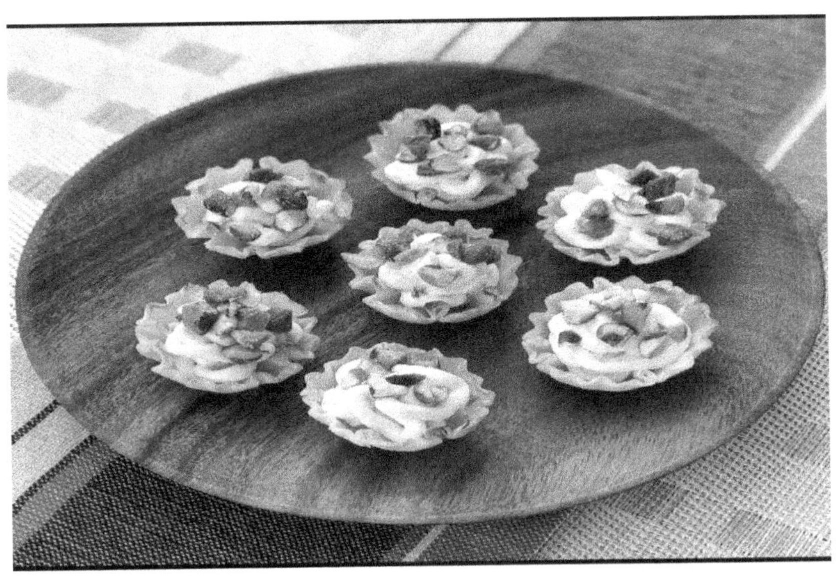

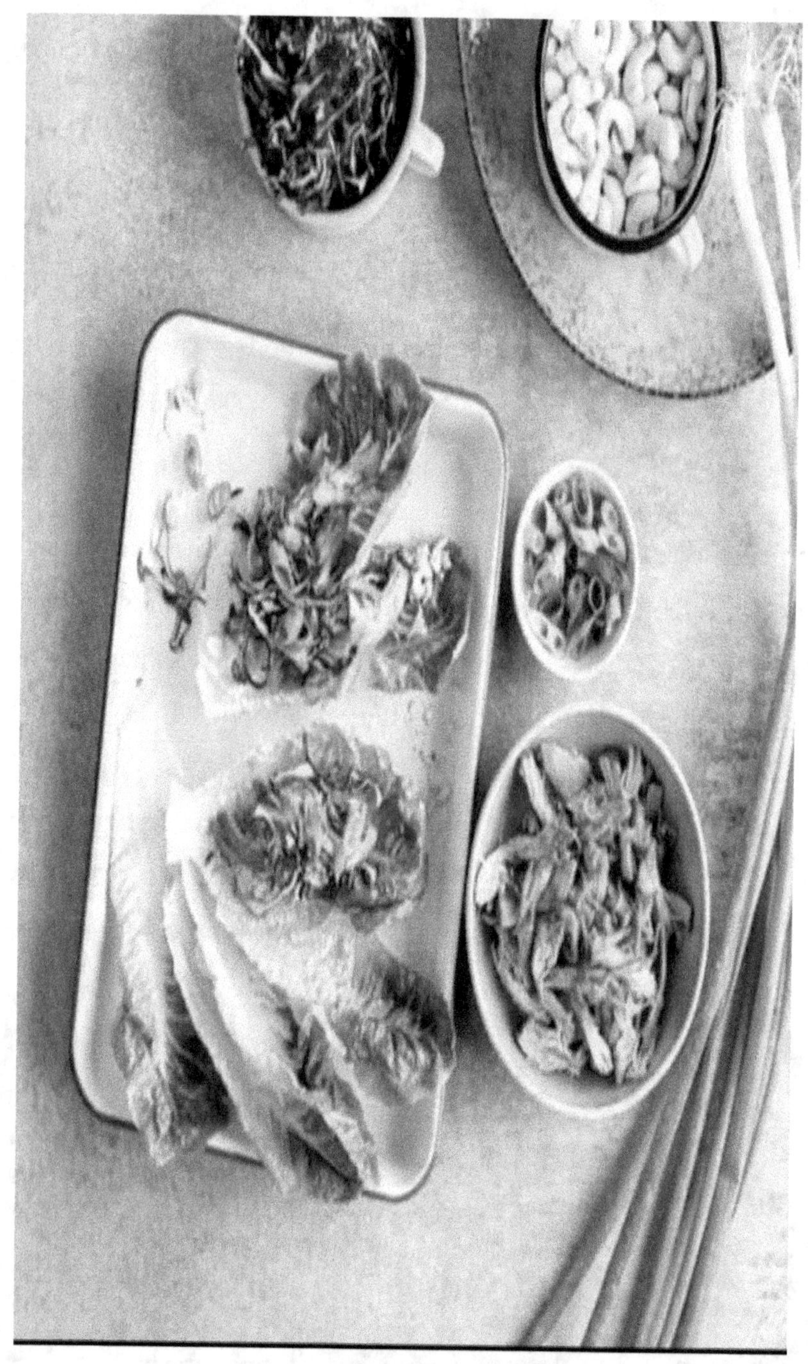

8. UNDERSTANDING AND MONITORING YOUR BLOOD SUGAR LEVELS

Effectively managing diabetes after 50 requires a solid understanding of how to monitor and interpret blood sugar levels. This section provides insights into the tools and techniques for blood sugar monitoring and the importance of keeping a detailed log of your food intake and glucose readings.

Tools and Techniques

Understanding Blood Sugar Monitoring Tools:

- **Glucose Meters:** These are the most common tools for checking blood sugar levels. They work by analyzing a small drop of your blood, usually taken from your fingertip.

- **Continuous Glucose Monitors (CGMs):** CGMs provide real-time readings of your glucose levels throughout the day and night. They involve a tiny sensor inserted under your skin.

- **A1C Test:** This blood test, typically done at a doctor's office, measures your average blood sugar levels over the past 2-3 months.

Techniques for Accurate Readings:

- **Consistent Timing:** Check your blood sugar at the same times each day, as advised by your healthcare provider, to track patterns and trends.

- **Proper Handling of Equipment:** Ensure your glucose meter and test strips are stored and handled correctly for accurate results.

- **Clean and Prepare the Site:** Clean your finger or the site where the blood will be drawn with soap and water to avoid contamination that might skew readings.

- **Record the Results:** Keeping a log of your results can help you and your healthcare provider make informed decisions about your diabetes management plan.

Understanding how to properly use these tools and techniques is vital for keeping track of your blood sugar levels and making necessary adjustments to your diet, exercise, and medication.

Keeping a Food and Blood Sugar Log

Maintaining a detailed food and blood sugar log is a critical aspect of managing diabetes effectively. This log can help you and your healthcare provider understand how different foods and activities affect your blood sugar levels, enabling more informed decisions regarding your diabetes management.

Key Elements of an Effective Log:

- **Record Food Intake:** Note down everything you eat and drink, along with portion sizes. Be as specific as possible.

- **Track Blood Sugar Levels:** Alongside your food log, record your blood sugar readings. Note the time of day and relation to meals (e.g., before breakfast, two hours after lunch).

- **Note Physical Activity:** Include details about your physical activity, including type, duration, and intensity. Exercise can significantly impact blood sugar levels.

- **Monitor How You Feel:** Pay attention to how you feel each day. Note any symptoms like fatigue, dizziness, or nausea, as they can be related to changes in blood sugar levels.

- **Include Other Relevant Information:** Record any additional factors that might affect your blood sugar, such as stress, illness, or changes in medication.

Benefits of Keeping a Log:

- **Identifies Patterns:** Helps recognize patterns and trends in blood sugar fluctuations in relation to diet and activity.

- **Informs Dietary Choices:** Assists in understanding which foods positively or negatively impact blood sugar control.

- **Enhances Communication with Healthcare Providers:** Provides valuable information to your healthcare team, allowing for more personalized diabetes care.

Tips for Effective Logging:

- **Be Consistent:** Make logging a daily habit for more accurate insights.

- **Use Tools That Work for You:** Whether it's a physical notebook, a digital app, or a spreadsheet, choose a method that's convenient and easy for you to maintain.

- **Review Regularly:** Periodically review your log to understand the effectiveness of your current diabetes management strategies and identify areas for improvement.

By diligently maintaining a food and blood sugar log, you can gain a deeper understanding of how your lifestyle affects your diabetes and make more informed choices to manage your condition effectively.

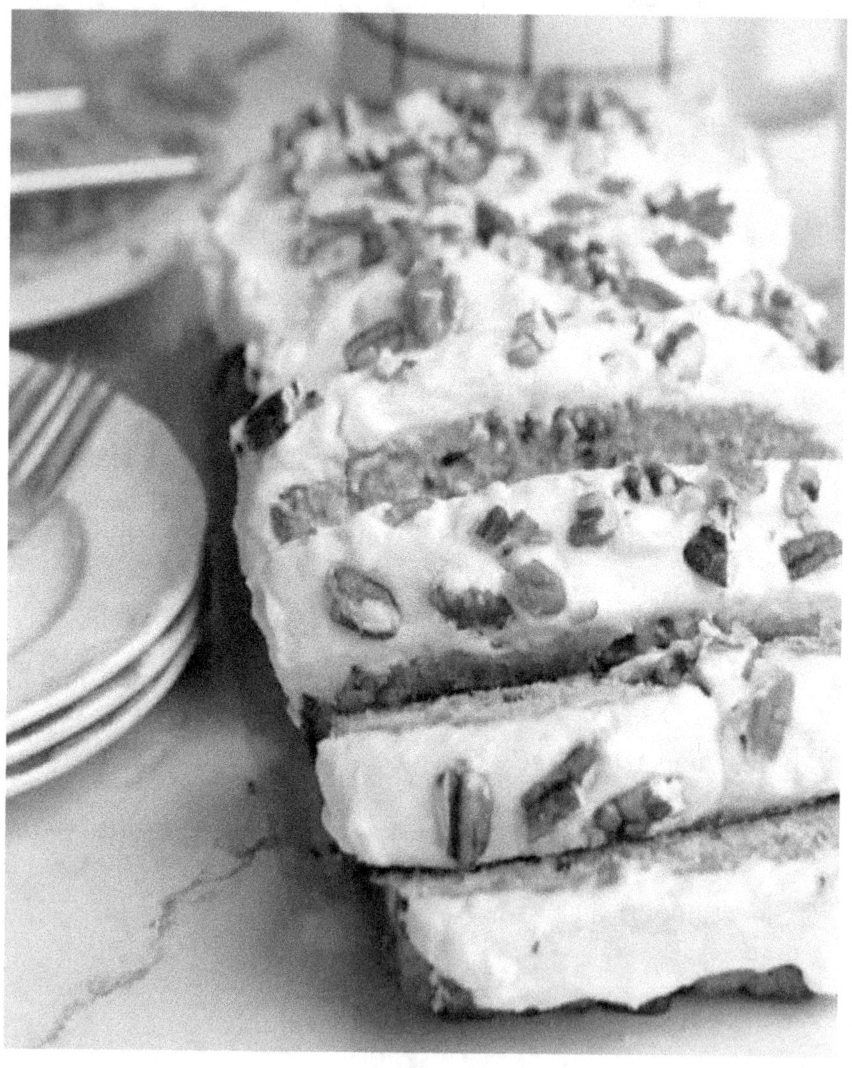

9. CONCLUSION

The journey through "Diabetic Diets Cookbook After 50" is not just about following recipes; it's about adopting a lifestyle that empowers you to manage your diabetes effectively. This conclusion wraps up the key elements of the book and reiterates the importance of a holistic approach to your health.

Empowering Yourself Through Diet and Lifestyle

Diet and Lifestyle as Tools for Empowerment:

- **Personal Responsibility:** Managing diabetes successfully involves taking personal responsibility for your daily choices. The foods you eat, the activities you engage in, and the way you manage stress all play a crucial role in controlling your diabetes.

- **Knowledge is Power:** Understanding the impact of different foods on your blood sugar levels, recognizing the importance of regular physical activity, and knowing how to manage stress are empowering. They equip you with the tools to take control of your diabetes, rather than letting it control you.

- **Customization is Key:** Everyone's body responds differently. Use the information and recipes in this book as a starting point, and tailor them to suit your individual needs and preferences.

- **Beyond Diet and Exercise:** Remember, managing diabetes is not just about diet and exercise. It's also about making informed decisions, staying educated about your condition, and maintaining regular communication with your healthcare providers.

Encouragement for the Journey:

- **Celebrate Small Victories:** Every healthy choice is a victory. Celebrate these moments, no matter how small.

- **Stay Positive and Patient:** Lifestyle changes take time to become habits. Be patient with yourself and stay positive.

- **Seek Support:** You're not alone in this journey. Family, friends, support groups, and healthcare professionals can provide support and guidance.

By empowering yourself through diet and lifestyle, you are taking a significant step towards better managing your diabetes and improving your overall quality of life.

Continuing Your Journey to Better Health

As you conclude "Diabetic Diets Cookbook After 50," remember that managing diabetes is an ongoing journey. It's a path of continuous learning, adapting, and improving. The journey to better health is not always linear; there will be successes and challenges. However, each step you take is a step towards a healthier, more fulfilling life.

Maintaining Momentum in Your Health Journey:

- **Stay Informed:** Keep up-to-date with the latest research and recommendations in diabetes care. Medical advice and dietary guidelines can evolve, so it's important to stay informed.

- **Regular Review and Adaptation:** Periodically review your diet, exercise routine, and blood sugar logs. Be prepared to adapt your strategies as your body and health needs change.

- **Long-Term Commitment:** Managing diabetes effectively is a long-term commitment. Embrace it as a permanent lifestyle change rather than a temporary fix.

- **Celebrate Your Progress:** Take time to acknowledge the progress you've made. Whether it's improved blood sugar levels, weight loss, or simply feeling better overall, these achievements are worth celebrating.

- **Share Your Knowledge:** Your experience can be invaluable to others. Consider sharing your journey and what you've learned with others who might be starting their own path to managing diabetes.

Looking to the Future:

- **Future Goals:** Set new health goals as you progress. This could be anything from trying new recipes to achieving certain blood sugar levels or fitness milestones.

- **Continual Support:** Continue to lean on your support network and healthcare team. They can provide motivation, advice, and help navigate any new challenges that arise.

Your journey to better health is a testament to your strength and commitment. Keep moving forward with the knowledge, skills, and habits you've developed. Remember, every step you take is an investment in your health and well-being.